NoMAD

Kidney Reboot, Cleaning out the Super Filter

NoMAD
Kidney Reboot, Cleaning out the Super Filter

What are the NoMAD Plans?

Developed by Dr Ash Kapoor, the NoMAD Plans represent a transformative approach to health and wellness that combines the wisdom of ancestral practices with contemporary medical insights. The name "NoMAD" not only suggests a journey through the intricate realm of health but also stands for its foundational principles: Nutritional Optimisation, Mindful Adaptation, and Detoxification.

At the heart of NoMAD is the 6R Framework—Restore, Release, Repair, Renew, Reframe, and Represent. This methodology addresses the root causes of illness, combats chronic inflammation, and cultivates authentic vitality, guiding individuals through a transformative process.

Tailored specifically to each individual, NoMAD journeys are meticulously crafted to rebalance the body, strengthen the mind, and rejuvenate overall health. By integrating ancestral practices with cutting-edge, innovative treatments—all under strict medical oversight—NoMAD Plans offer a personalised pathway to sustainable, long-lasting well-being that resonates with your unique life circumstances.

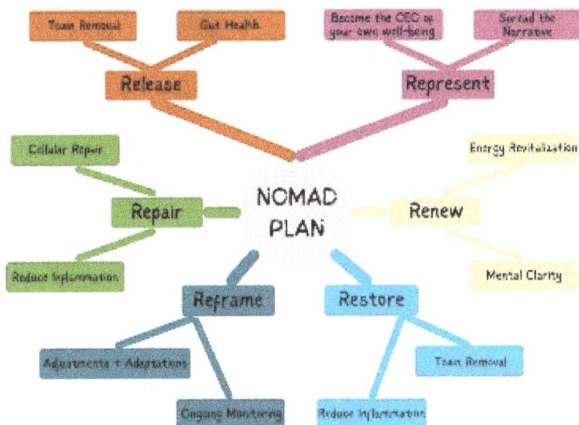

Levitas One:
"As Is In, As Is Out"

Reflecting the belief that our internal well-being is mirrored in our external environment. Founded by Dr Ash Kapoor, Levitas One serves as the vehicle for delivering NoMAD's treatment plans. It envisions a healthcare future where patients are at the centre of a fully integrated, multidisciplinary approach. Guided by Nomads 6 Rs— Restore, Release, Repair, Renew, Reframe, and Represent— Levitas One empowers self-care through personalised guidance and minimal intervention, promoting long-term health, balance, and sustainability.

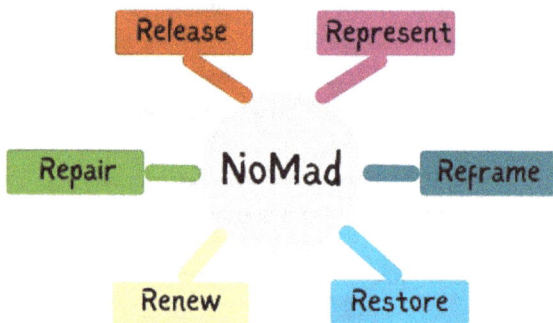

Release　　Represent

Repair　◄　NoMad　►　Reframe

Renew　　Restore

Contents

Preface

My name is Dr Ash Kapoor, and as a practising clinician with over 35 years of experience, I have witnessed firsthand the profound impact that detoxification can have on overall health. In particular, the role of the kidneys in maintaining the body's balance and vitality cannot be overstated. The kidneys act as the body's filtration system, removing waste products, regulating electrolytes, and balancing fluids. Yet, as critical as they are to our survival, many people overlook the importance of supporting kidney function until something goes wrong.

In today's world, kidney disease is on the rise, primarily due to modern lifestyles filled with processed foods, environmental toxins, chronic stress, and a sedentary existence. We live in a time when more people than ever before are being diagnosed with chronic kidney disease (CKD), and even more are experiencing suboptimal kidney function without realising it. This reality inspired me to explore ways to promote kidney health naturally, with the goal of preventing disease before it takes root.

Supporting kidney detoxification is one of the most effective strategies for prolonging healthy living. The kidneys, when functioning optimally, help remove toxins that accumulate from our diet, environment, and everyday metabolic processes. But like any other organ, they need care and support to continue operating at their best. Through simple yet powerful lifestyle changes—hydration, nutrition, exercise, herbal remedies, and stress management—we can take control of our kidney health and ensure that this vital organ continues to serve us well throughout our lives.

This book, *The Complete Guide to Kidney Cleansing: Holistic Health, Detoxification, and Longevity*, is a culmination of years of clinical observation, scientific research, and my dedication to empowering people with the tools they need to thrive. It is designed to educate and inspire readers of all ages to adopt preventive measures that protect their kidneys and enhance their overall well-being. Whether you are dealing with a kidney issue or simply looking to support long-term health, this book offers practical, evidence-based strategies for maintaining optimal kidney function.

The journey to a healthier life starts with understanding how to care for the body's essential systems. I hope the knowledge shared here will inspire you to act, improve your kidney health, and extend your longevity.

Introduction

Overview of Kidney Health and Detoxification

Your kidneys are two bean-shaped organs that play a fundamental role in maintaining overall health by filtering out waste, balancing fluids, regulating electrolytes, and controlling blood pressure. Despite their small size, these organs filter an astonishing 180 litres of blood daily, ensuring that waste products and excess fluids are removed from the body through urine. The kidneys not only remove metabolic byproducts like urea and creatinine but also help maintain the body's homeostasis, keeping the internal environment stable and balanced.

Kidneys are often overlooked when it comes to detoxification, as the liver and gut tend to take centre stage in most conversations about cleansing. However, the kidneys are integral to filtering out water-soluble toxins, medications, and excess nutrients. In the modern world, where environmental toxins, poor diets, and dehydration are common, our kidneys are working harder than ever before. The good news is that these resilient organs can be supported and protected through a combination of diet, lifestyle changes, and holistic therapies.

Detoxification is not only about removing harmful substances from the body; it is also about optimising your body's natural ability to eliminate waste. Kidney cleansing refers to a range of practices and interventions aimed at enhancing the kidneys' ability to detoxify the body, improving overall function, and reducing the risk of chronic diseases. This guide will introduce you to a holistic approach to kidney health, blending ancient wisdom with modern scientific understanding.

Why Kidney Cleansing is Important for Everyone

You don't have to have kidney disease or dysfunction to benefit from kidney cleansing. In fact, kidney health should be a priority for everyone—no matter your age or current health status. The kidneys perform essential functions that impact every aspect of your well-being, from maintaining electrolyte balance to producing hormones like erythropoietin, which stimulates red blood cell production. When the kidneys are not functioning optimally, it can lead to a range of health issues, including high blood pressure, fluid retention, fatigue, and more severe conditions like chronic kidney disease (CKD).

Over time, factors such as poor diet, chronic dehydration, excessive salt intake, and exposure to environmental toxins can put significant strain on your kidneys. By regularly supporting your kidneys through natural detoxification methods, you can help prevent long-term damage, maintain your energy levels, and protect your overall health.

Kidney cleansing involves a variety of strategies, from increasing hydration and consuming kidney-supportive foods to incorporating specific supplements, yoga practices, and alternative therapies like acupuncture and reflexology. These approaches can help improve kidney filtration, reduce the risk of kidney stones, and prevent other complications related to kidney health.

For younger individuals, kidney cleansing can help build a foundation for long-term health. At the same time, for middle-aged and older adults, it can be an important preventive measure to avoid common kidney-related issues such as hypertension and CKD. The idea is to support the kidneys' natural detoxification process, enhance their function, and ensure they remain resilient against the toxins and stressors encountered in daily life.

Critical Concepts for Readers of All Age Groups

This book is designed for individuals of all age groups, from young adults in their twenties to seniors in their seventies and beyond. Kidney health is crucial at every stage of life, and the earlier you start taking care of your kidneys, the better your chances of avoiding kidney dysfunction later in life.

For young adults in their 20s and 30s, the focus is on prevention. This period of life is about building healthy habits that protect your kidneys from long-term damage. Diet and hydration play a significant role in ensuring your kidneys function optimally. Avoiding excessive salt, processed foods, and sugar is vital, as is staying well-hydrated. Incorporating physical activity and being mindful of medications or substances that could harm the kidneys are essential steps toward lifelong kidney health.

For middle-aged adults in their 40s and 50s, kidney health becomes even more critical. This is often the stage where underlying health issues such as high blood pressure, diabetes, and weight gain can begin to impact the kidneys. If left unmanaged, these issues can increase the risk of CKD. At this stage, the book emphasises the importance of maintaining a balanced diet, regular exercise, and using targeted supplements to support kidney function. Practices such as intermittent fasting, which stimulates autophagy (the body's natural cellular cleanup process), can help the kidneys detoxify and regenerate.

For seniors, kidney function naturally declines with age, making it even more important to protect these vital organs. In your 60s, 70s, and beyond, strategies like hydration, kidney-supportive herbs (e.g., dandelion root, nettle), and medical interventions, such as IV hydration therapy, can be valuable. Regular screenings and being aware of the early signs of kidney dysfunction are essential for preventing complications. Seniors may also benefit from gentle yoga, acupuncture, and reflexology, which can support kidney health without overexerting the body.

The book will guide you through a variety of techniques and lifestyle changes tailored to your age and current health status. You'll learn how to recognise the early signs of kidney dysfunction, how to prevent kidney problems before they arise, and how to improve your kidney health at any age. Whether you are young and healthy, dealing with early signs of kidney issues, or managing a chronic condition like CKD, this guide will provide practical, actionable advice that you can start implementing today.

Conclusion

By the end of this book, you'll have a solid understanding of how your kidneys work and what steps you can take to cleanse, support, and protect them. Whether you are exploring natural methods for kidney detoxification, looking for preventive measures to maintain kidney health, or seeking to manage an existing condition, the practices and insights shared in this guide will empower you to take control of your kidney health.

We will explore holistic approaches such as diet, exercise, herbs, and alternative therapies alongside modern medical interventions that can enhance kidney function. With real-life case studies, scientific explanations, and practical tips, this book is your comprehensive resource for supporting one of your body's most essential systems—the kidneys.

Let's dive into the journey of kidney health and longevity!

Summary: Introduction

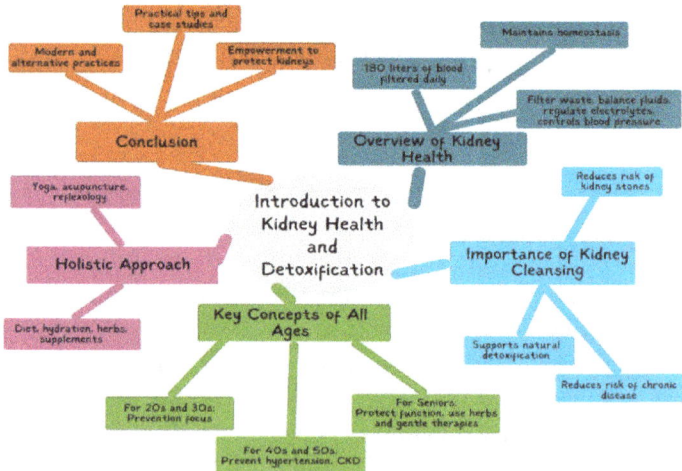

Chapter 1
Understanding the Kidneys

Anatomy of the Kidneys in Simple Terms

The kidneys are two small, bean-shaped organs located on either side of your spine, just below the rib cage. Each kidney is roughly the size of a fist. Despite their modest size, they perform a range of vital functions that are essential to your overall health.

The outer layer of the kidney is called the **renal cortex**, while the inner part is known as the **renal medulla**. Inside each kidney, there are about a million tiny structures called **nephrons**—the functional units that filter your blood. Nephrons are responsible for removing waste, excess water, and unwanted substances from the bloodstream. Each nephron consists of a **glomerulus** (a bundle of tiny blood vessels) and a **tubule** (a long tube through which filtered substances pass).

Blood flows into the kidneys through the **renal arteries**, where it is filtered by the glomeruli. Once filtered, waste and excess substances are turned into urine, which is passed through the tubules, collected in the **renal pelvis**, and transported to the bladder via two tubes called **ureters**. Clean, filtered blood leaves the kidneys through the **renal veins** and returns to the rest of the body.

Although the kidneys are primarily known for their role in urine production, they also help maintain the balance of important substances such as electrolytes (sodium, potassium, calcium) and regulate blood pressure by manageing fluid balance. Additionally, the kidneys produce hormones, including **erythropoietin**, which stimulates red blood cell production, and **renin**, which helps regulate blood pressure.

The Role of Kidneys in the Body's Detoxification System

The primary function of the kidneys is to filter the blood, removing waste products and excess substances while maintaining the body's balance of water and electrolytes. Every day, your kidneys filter about 50 gallons (180 litres) of blood, extracting harmful toxins, waste products, and excess water, which are then excreted as urine.

The detoxification process in the kidneys happens in three key steps:

1. **Filtration:** Blood flows through the glomeruli, where waste products such as urea (a byproduct of protein metabolism), creatinine (a byproduct of muscle metabolism), and excess ions (such as sodium and potassium) are filtered out of the bloodstream.

2. **Reabsorption:** As the filtrate passes through the nephron tubules, essential substances like glucose, water, and electrolytes are reabsorbed back into the bloodstream, ensuring that the body retains what it needs for normal functioning.

3. **Secretion:** Finally, certain waste products and excess ions are secreted into the tubules for excretion. The result is urine, which is sent to the bladder to be stored and eventually expelled from the body.

In addition to waste removal, the kidneys play a critical role in regulating the body's **pH balance** by controlling the levels of hydrogen and bicarbonate ions. They also help detoxify various substances, including medications, alcohol, and environmental toxins, by filtering these compounds from the blood and facilitating their removal from the body.

Analogy: The Kidneys as the Body's Water Treatment Plant

One of the best ways to understand the kidneys' function is by thinking of them as the body's water treatment plant. Just as a water treatment facility filters out pollutants, debris, and harmful chemicals to provide clean water, your kidneys filter your blood to remove waste and maintain the body's internal environment.

Imagine a stream of water flowing into a treatment plant. The water contains both harmful substances (like pollutants) and essential elements (like minerals). The treatment plant's job is to remove the harmful substances while retaining the clean water and important minerals. In this analogy, your blood is the water, and the kidneys act as the filtration system.

Just like a water treatment plant must work efficiently to ensure that only clean water passes through to homes and businesses, your kidneys must continuously filter your blood to ensure your body remains free of harmful toxins. If the treatment plant fails, harmful substances can build up in the water, making it dangerous to drink. Similarly, suppose your kidneys aren't functioning properly. In that case, toxins and waste products can accumulate in your blood, leading to serious health problems.

This analogy helps illustrate how essential the kidneys are to maintaining a clean and healthy internal environment. Much like how we take clean water for granted, many people don't think about their kidneys until they stop working efficiently. Understanding this comparison makes it easier to appreciate the importance of keeping your kidneys healthy.

Common Kidney Problems and How to Recognise Them

Kidney problems are often referred to as "silent" because they can develop slowly over time without noticeable symptoms. However, certain warning signs can indicate that your kidneys may not be functioning correctly. Here are some of the most common kidney problems and the symptoms to watch for:

1. Chronic Kidney Disease (CKD):

CKD is a gradual loss of kidney function over time. Early stages of CKD often have no symptoms, but as the disease progresses, you may notice:

a. Fatigue and weakness
b. Swelling in the legs, ankles, or feet (oedema)
c. Shortness of breath
d. Difficulty concentrating
e. High blood pressure that is hard to control
f. Changes in urination (more or less frequent, foamy urine, or blood in the urine)

Prevention Tip: Regular checkups and blood tests (such as measuring creatinine levels and glomerular filtration rate, or GFR) can detect CKD early, allowing for better management.

2. Kidney Stones:

Kidney stones are hard deposits of minerals and salts that form inside the kidneys. They can be extremely painful as they pass through the urinary tract. Common symptoms include:

a. Severe pain in the back, sides, or abdomen
b. Painful urination
c. Pink, red, or brown urine (indicating blood in the urine)
d. Nausea or vomiting
e. Urgent and frequent need to urinate

Prevention Tip: Staying well-hydrated and reducing sodium intake can lower the risk of developing kidney stones.

3. Urinary Tract Infections (UTIs):

UTIs occur when bacteria enter the urinary tract, leading to infection. If left untreated, the infection can spread to the kidneys (pyelonephritis), causing more severe symptoms, such as:

a. Pain or burning sensation when urinating
b. Cloudy, foul-smelling, or bloody urine
c. Fever and chills
d. Pain in the lower back or sides

Prevention Tip: Drinking plenty of water and practising good hygiene can help prevent UTIs.

4. Acute Kidney Injury (AKI):

AKI is a sudden loss of kidney function, often due to dehydration, injury, or exposure to toxic substances. Symptoms include:

a.   Decreased urine output
b.   Swelling in the legs or feet
c.   Fatigue or confusion
d.   Shortness of breath
e.   Chest pain or pressure

Prevention Tip: Avoiding overuse of medications that are hard on the kidneys (such as NSAIDs) and staying hydrated can reduce the risk of AKI.

5. Polycystic Kidney Disease (PKD):

PKD is a genetic disorder where clusters of cysts form in the kidneys, causing them to enlarge and lose function over time. Symptoms include:

a.   High blood pressure
b.   Pain or heaviness in the back or sides
c.   Blood in the urine
d.   Kidney stones
e.   Kidney failure (in severe cases)

Prevention Tip: While PKD is genetic and cannot be prevented, manageing blood pressure and monitoring kidney function can slow the progression of the disease.

Conclusion

Understanding the anatomy and function of the kidneys is the first step toward appreciating the crucial role they play in detoxification and overall health. By recognising common kidney problems and taking proactive steps to support your kidneys through hydration, a healthy diet, and regular check-ups, you can help maintain optimal kidney function throughout your life. Whether you are dealing with kidney issues or simply looking to prevent them, this chapter lays the foundation for a deeper understanding of how your kidneys work and why they are vital to your well-being.

Summary: Understanding the Kidneys

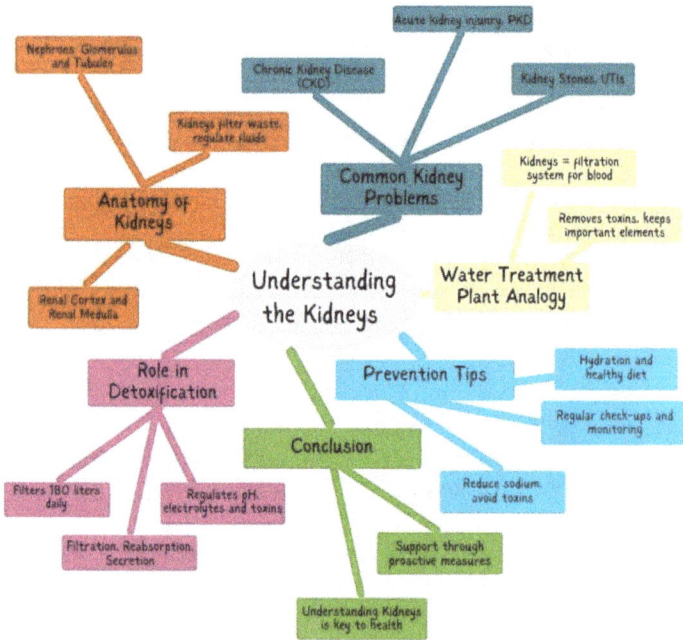

Chapter 2
Autophagy – The Body's Cellular Cleanup Mechanism

What is Autophagy?

Autophagy is a natural process in the body where cells break down and recycle their own components. The term "autophagy" comes from the Greek words **"auto"** meaning self, and **"phagy"** meaning eating, so autophagy literally means "self-eating." While this may sound alarming, autophagy is a beneficial and essential function that allows cells to clear out damaged or dysfunctional components and regenerate healthy cellular structures.

This cellular cleanup process is crucial for maintaining overall health, as it helps to eliminate damaged proteins, worn-out organelles, and other cellular debris that could accumulate and cause harm. Autophagy acts as a quality control mechanism, ensuring that only the healthiest cells continue functioning optimally. This is especially important in tissues like the kidneys, which are responsible for filtering waste and toxins from the blood.

At its core, autophagy is a survival mechanism, allowing the body to efficiently recycle parts of the cell that are no longer functioning well and use them for energy or as building blocks for new cellular structures. When the body is under stress, such as during periods of fasting or intense exercise, autophagy is activated, providing the body with essential nutrients and clearing out harmful materials.

How Autophagy Helps with Kidney Health and Detoxification

The kidneys, like all organs, undergo cellular wear and tear over time. Cells in the kidneys are constantly exposed to various toxins, metabolic waste products, and oxidative stress due to their filtration role. Autophagy plays a significant role in maintaining kidney health by clearing out damaged cells and proteins preventing the accumulation of waste that can lead to cellular dysfunction.

Protection Against Oxidative Stress: The kidneys are exposed to oxidative stress, which can damage cells and impair their function. Oxidative stress occurs when there's an imbalance between free radicals (unstable molecules) and the body's ability to neutralise them with antioxidants. Autophagy helps reduce oxidative stress by clearing out damaged mitochondria (the powerhouses of cells), which are a primary source of free radicals. By removing dysfunctional mitochondria and replacing them with healthier ones, autophagy ensures that kidney cells continue to function optimally.

Prevention of Kidney Disease: Autophagy is critical in preventing chronic kidney diseases like **diabetic nephropathy** and **glomerulonephritis,** conditions that lead to long-term kidney damage. In the early stages of kidney disease, autophagy helps reduce inflammation and fibrosis (scarring) by degrading damaged proteins and cellular debris that contribute to disease progression. Studies have shown that insufficient autophagy can accelerate the progression of kidney disease by allowing the buildup of harmful proteins and promoting fibrosis.

Detoxification Support: Autophagy also aids in the detoxification process. When harmful substances, such as medications, environmental toxins, or metabolic byproducts, accumulate in the kidneys, they can lead to cellular damage. Autophagy breaks down these toxic substances at the cellular level, ensuring they are processed and removed efficiently. This is particularly important when the kidneys are under stress from high toxin loads, as autophagy helps protect kidney cells from the long-term effects of toxicity.

Prevention of Kidney Ageing: As we age, the efficiency of autophagy naturally declines, leading to the accumulation of cellular waste and damaged proteins in the kidneys. This can contribute to age-related kidney dysfunction. Supporting autophagy through lifestyle interventions can help mitigate these effects, slowing the natural ageing process of the kidneys and preserving their function over time.

How to Stimulate Autophagy (Intermittent Fasting, Exercise, etc.)

Stimulating autophagy is an effective way to enhance cellular health and support kidney function. There are several natural methods for activating autophagy, and the following are some of the most well-researched approaches:

1. **Intermittent Fasting:** One of the most effective ways to stimulate autophagy is through intermittent fasting, which involves cycling between periods of eating and fasting. When the body enters a fasted state, energy and nutrient levels drop, prompting cells to initiate autophagy as a way to recycle their internal components for energy. Research has shown that fasting for 16 to 24 hours can significantly activate autophagy, particularly in the kidneys. This is why intermittent fasting is considered a powerful tool for promoting cellular repair and longevity.

   Example Protocol:

   a. **16:8 method:** Fast for 16 hours each day, with an 8-hour window for eating.
   b. **24-hour fast:** Once or twice a week, fast for a full 24 hours to deeply stimulate autophagy.

2. **Exercise:** Exercise is another powerful activator of autophagy, particularly in the kidneys and other organs. When you exercise, your body experiences mild stress, and cells begin to break down and recycle damaged components to maintain energy balance. Exercise also stimulates the production of mitochondria, improving the overall health and function of kidney cells. Regular aerobic exercise, such as running, swimming, or cycling, has been shown to enhance autophagy, particularly when performed at moderate to high intensity.

Best Practices:

a. Engage in moderate aerobic exercise for at least 30 minutes, 5 times a week.

b. Incorporate resistance training to promote muscle health and cellular repair.

3. **Caloric Restriction:** Reducing caloric intake while maintaining essential nutrients is another way to promote autophagy. Caloric restriction has been shown to increase lifespan and improve kidney function by reducing the accumulation of damaged proteins and enhancing cellular repair mechanisms. This approach mimics the effects of fasting and helps maintain cellular health over the long term.

    How to Implement:

    a. Reduce daily caloric intake by 20-30% while maintaining adequate intake of vitamins, minerals, and protein.

    b. Consider practising caloric restriction a few days each week to avoid chronic energy deficits.

4. **Autophagy-Boosting Compounds:** Certain compounds and supplements can enhance autophagy. For example, **resveratrol** (found in red grapes and berries), **curcumin** (found in turmeric), and **green tea** have been shown to stimulate autophagy by activating specific pathways in the body. These natural substances help protect the kidneys from oxidative stress and promote healthy cellular turnover.

    Recommended Supplements:

    a. **Resveratrol:** 200-500 mg/day

    b. **Curcumin:** 500-1000 mg/day

    c. **Green tea extract:** 500-1000 mg/day

5. **Ketogenic Diet:** A ketogenic (low-carb, high-fat) diet has been shown to mimic fasting by lowering glucose levels and increasing ketone production, which can activate autophagy. The diet forces the body to rely on fat for fuel, which triggers the breakdown and recycling of damaged cellular components. A ketogenic diet has also been shown to support kidney health by reducing inflammation and oxidative stress.

Case Study: Stimulating Autophagy for Kidney Health in a 45-Year-Old Office Worker

Background:

John, a 45-year-old office worker, had been experiencing signs of early kidney dysfunction, including elevated creatinine levels and occasional fatigue. He had a sedentary lifestyle, often sitting for long hours, and a diet high in processed foods. His doctor warned him that if he didn't make lifestyle changes, he could be at risk for chronic kidney disease (CKD). Seeking a more natural approach to improve his kidney health, John decided to explore ways to stimulate autophagy.

Intervention:

John adopted a combination of intermittent fasting and regular exercise to activate autophagy and support his kidneys. He started by practising the **16:8 intermittent fasting method,** fasting for 16 hours each day and eating within an 8-hour window. This allowed his body to enter a fasted state, triggering autophagy and cellular repair. He also began incorporating moderate aerobic exercise, walking for 30 minutes daily, and gradually adding cycling to his routine.

In addition to fasting and exercise, John adjusted his diet to reduce processed foods and added more kidney-friendly foods such as berries, leafy greens, and healthy fats like olive oil. He also started taking supplements like **resveratrol** and **green tea extract** to further support autophagy.

Outcome:

After three months of these interventions, John saw significant improvements in his kidney health. His creatinine levels dropped, and his energy levels improved. He reported feeling more alert and less fatigued during the day. His doctor noted that his kidney function had stabilised, and there was no further indication of progression toward CKD.

John's experience demonstrates how autophagy can be stimulated through simple lifestyle changes, providing a powerful tool for enhancing kidney health. By incorporating intermittent fasting, exercise, and autophagy-boosting compounds, he was able to take control of his health and improve his kidney function naturally.

Conclusion

Autophagy is the body's natural way of cleaning out damaged cells and regenerating healthier ones, making it a crucial process for maintaining kidney health. By stimulating autophagy through intermittent fasting, exercise, caloric restriction, and the use of natural compounds, you can support your kidneys in their vital role of detoxification and waste elimination. Whether you are looking to prevent kidney issues or improve your current kidney function, autophagy offers a powerful, scientifically-backed way to enhance cellular health and promote long-term well-being.

Summary: Autophagy – The Body's Cellular Cleanup Mechanism

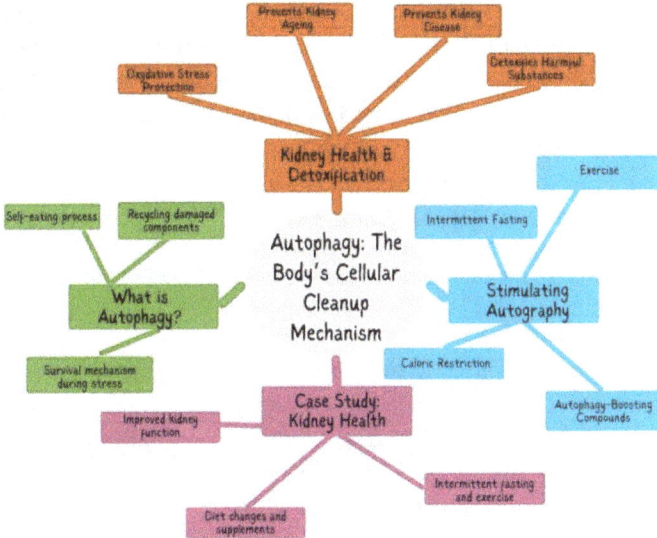

The diagram is a mind map titled "Autophagy: The Body's Cellular Cleanup Mechanism" with the following branches:

- **Kidney Health & Detoxification**: Prevents Kidney Ageing, Prevents Kidney Disease, Detoxifies Harmful Substances, Oxidative Stress Protection
- **What is Autophagy?**: Self-eating process, Recycling damaged components, Survival mechanism during stress
- **Stimulating Autography**: Exercise, Intermittent Fasting, Caloric Restriction, Autophagy-Boosting Compounds
- **Case Study: Kidney Health**: Improved kidney function, Diet changes and supplements, Intermittent fasting and exercise

Chapter 3
Historical Perspectives on Kidney Cleansing

The quest for kidney health is not a modern pursuit. Ancient civilisations understood the importance of the kidneys for overall health and incorporated various techniques for maintaining their function. From the Egyptians to the Greeks and Romans, and through to the holistic systems of Ayurveda and Traditional Chinese Medicine (TCM), kidney cleansing practices have long been an essential component of health and well-being. The knowledge passed down from these ancient traditions continues to influence modern wellness, offering time-tested approaches to support and protect the kidneys.

Ancient Egyptian, Greek, and Roman Practices for Kidney Health

The ancient Egyptians were pioneers in the field of medicine, and their medical papyri provide valuable insights into how they viewed the body's organs, including the kidneys. Although their understanding of anatomy was limited compared to today, the Egyptians recognised the importance of the kidneys in maintaining the body's fluid balance and in the excretion of waste. They used herbal concoctions to promote diuresis (increased urination) and alleviate symptoms of kidney dysfunction, often resorting to natural remedies like celery, juniper, and parsley. These herbs, which are known for their diuretic properties, helped to cleanse the kidneys and maintain urinary tract health.

Moving westward, the Greeks and Romans, deeply influenced by the medical teachings of Hippocrates and later Galen, expanded upon the role of the kidneys. Hippocrates, often referred to as the "Father of Medicine," believed that kidney function was closely tied to overall health and well-being. He viewed the kidneys as responsible for filtering excess fluids from the body and maintaining humoral balance, the ancient belief that health was determined by the balance of bodily fluids, or humours.

Galen, a prominent Greek physician during the Roman Empire, further advanced the understanding of kidney health. He documented in great detail how the kidneys played a crucial role in filtering blood and eliminating toxins from the body. Galen also suggested that certain foods and herbs could support kidney function. Fennel, asparagus, and cucumber, which were commonly used in Roman diets, were considered particularly beneficial for the kidneys due to their ability to promote urination and reduce water retention. These ancient Greek and Roman practices focused on diet and herbal remedies, recognising that a healthy lifestyle supported proper kidney function and longevity.

Traditional Practices in Ayurveda and Traditional Chinese Medicine (TCM)

Both Ayurveda and Traditional Chinese Medicine (TCM) have rich histories of treating the kidneys holistically, with an emphasis on balancing the body's energies and maintaining overall health. These ancient medical systems continue to inform modern approaches to kidney health.

In Ayurveda, the kidneys are seen as part of the body's **Mutravaha Srotas** (urinary system) and are crucial for regulating water and electrolyte balance. Ayurvedic texts highlight the importance of keeping the kidneys and urinary tract free from impurities to prevent disease and enhance vitality. Key herbs in Ayurveda for kidney health include **Punarnava**, which is well-known for its diuretic and anti-inflammatory properties, **Gokshura**, used to support kidney function and maintain healthy urination, and **Shilajit**, a rejuvenative substance believed to strengthen the kidneys and support overall detoxification.

Ayurvedic practitioners also advocate for the practice of **Panchakarma**, a detoxification and rejuvenation process that includes dietary changes, herbal treatments, oil massages, and cleansing enemas to remove accumulated toxins from the body. Through these techniques, Ayurveda emphasises a preventive approach, aiming to strengthen kidney function before imbalances manifest as disease.

Traditional Chinese Medicine (TCM) similarly views the kidneys as one of the most vital organs, governing the body's **Jing** (essence) and **Qi** (energy). In TCM, the kidneys are considered the source of life force, influencing everything from longevity to reproductive health. The kidneys are seen as the body's "water element," managing the body's fluids and excreting waste. **Kidney Yin** and **Kidney Yang** represent the balance of cooling and warming energies within the body, and any disharmony between the two can lead to kidney-related ailments.

To support kidney health, TCM practitioners often prescribe **Rehmannia**, a herb used to nourish Kidney Yin, and **Cordyceps**, a fungus believed to restore Kidney Yang and promote overall vitality. Acupuncture is also frequently used in TCM to stimulate specific meridian points related to the kidneys, balancing the body's energy and promoting detoxification. By aligning the kidneys with the body's broader energy system, TCM offers a comprehensive approach to kidney cleansing and well-being.

Lessons from the Past: How Ancient Kidney Cleansing Influences Modern Wellness

To further expand on the significance of these historical kidney cleansing practices, it is important to delve deeper into how these ancient systems approached the prevention of kidney-related diseases. In both Ayurveda and Traditional Chinese Medicine (TCM), prevention has always been emphasised over treatment, a perspective that resonates strongly with today's movement towards preventive health care.

In Ayurveda, one of the fundamental concepts is **Ojas**, the essence of vitality and immunity, which is believed to be deeply connected to kidney health. When the kidneys function optimally,

Ojas is said to be in balance, promoting resilience and longevity. Ancient Ayurvedic texts encouraged not only the use of herbs and dietary practices for kidney support but also the integration of **meditation** and **yogic breathing exercises (Pranayama)** to reduce stress—a known contributor to kidney strain and disease. Modern research now acknowledges that chronic stress elevates cortisol levels, which can contribute to high blood pressure, a leading cause of kidney disease. Practices that reduce stress, such as meditation and yoga, align with ancient Ayurvedic wisdom that sought to maintain harmony between the mind and body for optimal organ function.

In TCM, **balance between the Yin and Yang** forces within the body was seen as key to preventing disease. The kidneys, considered the storehouse of Jing (the essence of life), were believed to be particularly susceptible to imbalances caused by overwork, poor diet, and emotional stress. Ancient Chinese physicians recommended seasonal detoxifications, herbal tonics, and acupuncture sessions to support kidney vitality throughout the year. This idea of tuning into seasonal rhythms and making adjustments to diet and lifestyle based on environmental changes is gaining popularity in modern wellness, particularly in the fields of integrative and functional medicine.

Modern research now validates many of the herbal remedies used by ancient cultures. For example, scientific studies have confirmed that **Punarnava** has diuretic properties that help flush excess water from the kidneys, making it an effective remedy for managing water retention and kidney health. Similarly, **Cordyceps** has gained popularity as a supplement that not only supports kidney function but also enhances athletic performance and boosts energy levels—properties that ancient Chinese practitioners were aware of centuries ago.

Today's holistic practitioners often integrate these ancient practices with modern medicine, combining herbs like **dandelion**, **nettle**, and **turmeric**—which are known for their ability to support kidney health—with advances in medical diagnostics. The fusion of ancient wisdom and modern science offers a comprehensive framework for kidney cleansing that is accessible to individuals seeking to improve their health naturally.

The primary lesson from ancient civilisations is that kidney health requires consistent care and attention. The kidneys are not just vital for detoxification but also for maintaining the balance of the body's entire internal environment. Whether through diet, herbal remedies, or mindful practices like yoga and acupuncture, supporting kidney function is key to living a long, healthy, and vibrant life.

Conclusion

Ancient civilisations, from the Egyptians to the Greeks and Romans, as well as holistic systems like Ayurveda and Traditional Chinese Medicine, recognised the essential role of the kidneys in maintaining health and vitality. Their focus on natural remedies, diet, and balance offers valuable insights for modern wellness practices. As we face rising levels of chronic kidney disease and environmental toxins, the lessons from the past can guide us toward a healthier future. By combining ancient wisdom with modern approaches, we can better support our kidneys, promote detoxification, and enhance our overall well-being.

Summary:

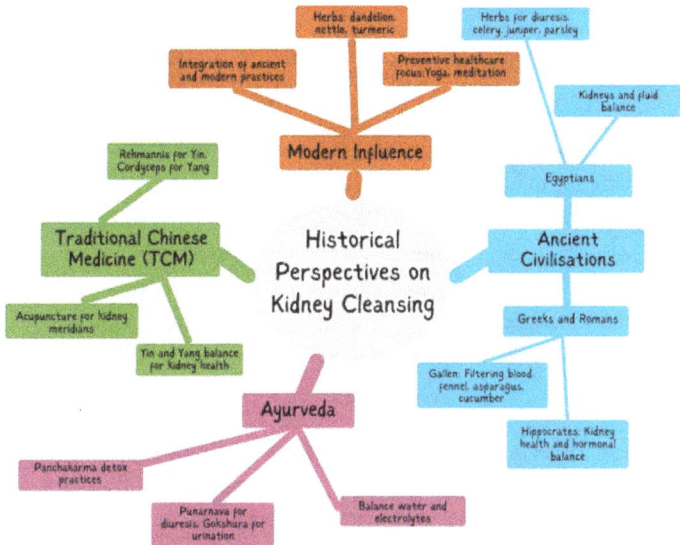

Chapter 4
Yoga for Kidney Health and Detoxification

Introduction to Yoga and Its Benefits for Kidney
Function

Yoga is an ancient practice that combines physical postures (asanas), breathing techniques (pranayama), and meditation to promote overall health and well-being. In recent years, yoga has gained recognition not only as a practice for mental clarity and flexibility but also for its powerful effects on internal organs, including the kidneys. Yoga's ability to stimulate blood flow, improve oxygenation, and reduce stress makes it an excellent tool for supporting kidney function and detoxification.

The kidneys, like other organs, rely on proper circulation and oxygenation to function optimally. Yoga postures specifically designed to target the abdominal and lower back regions can improve blood flow to the kidneys, helping them filter waste more efficiently. Additionally, yoga helps reduce stress, which can have a profound impact on kidney health. Chronic stress increases cortisol levels, which can raise blood pressure and damage the kidneys over time. Yoga helps lower cortisol and regulate blood pressure, protecting the kidneys from stress-related harm.

Moreover, yoga aids in detoxification by stimulating the lymphatic system, which helps the body clear out toxins and waste products. This, combined with its ability to calm the nervous system and promote relaxation, makes yoga a holistic approach to kidney health.

Key Yoga Postures (Asanas) to Stimulate Kidney Detox

Certain yoga postures are particularly beneficial for improving kidney health. These poses work by enhancing circulation, stretching the muscles around the kidneys, and supporting the detoxification process. Here are some key asanas that specifically target the kidneys:

1.   Ardha Matsyendrasana (Half Lord of the Fishes Pose)

Ardha Matsyendrasana is a spinal twist that stretches the muscles around the kidneys and promotes circulation to the abdominal organs. Twisting poses like this one help compress and then release the kidneys, encouraging fresh blood flow and improved detoxification.

How to Perform:

a.   Sit on the floor with your legs extended in front of you.
b.   Bend your right knee and place your foot on the outside of your left thigh.
c.   Place your left elbow on the outside of your right knee and twist your torso to the right.
d.   Hold for 30 seconds to a minute, breathing deeply, then switch sides.

2.   Bhujangasana (Cobra Pose)

Cobra Pose strengthens the muscles of the lower back and stimulates blood flow to the kidneys. It also opens up the chest, improving lung capacity and oxygenation of the blood, which benefits kidney function.

How to Perform:

a.   Lie face down on the mat with your hands placed under your shoulders.
b.   Press through your palms to lift your chest off the ground, keeping your elbows close to your body.
c.   Engage your lower back muscles, lifting your chest higher while keeping your pelvis on the floor.

d.   Hold for 20-30 seconds, breathing deeply.

3.   Paschimottanasana (Seated Forward Bend)

This forward-bending pose stretches the lower back and stimulates the kidneys by compressing the abdominal area. It encourages relaxation and helps reduce stress, both of which are essential for maintaining kidney health.

How to Perform:

a.   Sit with your legs extended straight in front of you.
b.   Inhale, lengthen your spine and exhale as you fold forward, reaching for your feet or ankles.
c.   Keep your back straight and avoid rounding the spine.
d.   Hold the pose for 1-2 minutes, breathing deeply.

4.   Setu Bandhasana (Bridge Pose)

Bridge Pose strengthens the lower back and stimulates circulation to the kidneys by gently compressing the abdomen. It also opens up the chest, improving breathing and oxygenation.

How to Perform:

a.   Lie on your back with your knees bent and feet flat on the floor, hip-width apart.
b.   Press through your feet and lift your hips towards the ceiling.
c.   Clasp your hands underneath your back and press your arms into the floor.
d.   Hold for 30 seconds to a minute, then release and lower your hips back to the ground.

5.   Supta Baddha Konasana (Reclining Bound Angle Pose)

This restorative pose opens the hips and relaxes the lower body, promoting relaxation and stress relief, which are vital for maintaining kidney health. It also encourages circulation in the pelvic region, supporting kidney function.

How to Perform:

a.   Lie on your back and bring the soles of your feet together, allowing your knees to fall open.

b.   Place a bolster or folded blankets under your knees for support if needed.

c.   Rest your arms by your sides, palms facing up, and breathe deeply.

d.   Stay in this pose for 3-5 minutes, allowing your body to relax fully.

Breathing Exercises (Pranayama) for Kidney Support

In addition to physical postures, breathing exercises (pranayama) are an integral part of yoga practice and have a direct impact on kidney function. Deep, mindful breathing increases oxygen intake, which improves blood flow to the kidneys and enhances their ability to filter waste. Here are two powerful pranayama techniques that can support kidney health:

1.   Nadi Shodhana (Alternate Nostril Breathing)

Nadi Shodhana is a calming breathing technique that balances the body's energy and reduces stress. By lowering stress levels and promoting relaxation, this pranayama helps protect the kidneys from the damaging effects of chronic stress and high blood pressure.

How to Perform:

a.   Sit comfortably with your spine straight and shoulders relaxed.

b.   Close your right nostril with your thumb and inhale deeply through your left nostril.

c.   Close your left nostril with your ring finger, release your thumb, and exhale through your right nostril.

d.   Inhale through your right nostril, close it with your thumb, and exhale through your left nostril.

e.   Repeat for 5-10 minutes, focusing on smooth, even breaths.

2. Kapalabhati (Skull Shining Breath)

Kapalabhati is an energising breathing exercise that involves forceful exhalations to cleanse the lungs and improve circulation. This pranayama stimulates the abdominal organs, including the kidneys, and helps detoxify the body.

How to Perform:

a. Sit comfortably with your spine straight and hands resting on your knees.
b. Take a deep breath in, and as you exhale, forcefully contract your abdominal muscles, expelling the air through your nostrils in short bursts.
c. Inhale passively between exhalations, allowing your lungs to fill naturally.
d. Continue for 1-2 minutes, then take a deep breath and relax.

Case Study: How a 60-Year-Old Man Improved Kidney Function through Yoga

Background: Mark, a 60-year-old man, had been struggling with mild kidney dysfunction for several years. He was diagnosed with stage 2 chronic kidney disease (CKD). He was advised by his doctor to make lifestyle changes to improve his kidney function. Mark had a sedentary job and a high-stress lifestyle, both of which were contributing factors to his declining kidney health. Although his doctor recommended medication to manage his blood pressure, Mark wanted to explore natural ways to support his kidneys.

Intervention: Mark began practising yoga three times a week, focusing on gentle asanas and breathing exercises that specifically targeted kidney health. His yoga routine included **Ardha Matsyendrasana (Half Lord of the Fishes Pose), Bhujangasana (Cobra Pose),** and **Setu Bandhasana (Bridge Pose)** to stimulate circulation and improve detoxification. He also incorporated **Nadi**

Shodhana (Alternate Nostril Breathing) into his daily practice to reduce stress and regulate his blood pressure.

Mark also made dietary adjustments, increasing his water intake and reducing his consumption of processed foods while continuing to monitor his blood pressure regularly.

Outcome: After three months of consistent yoga practice, Mark's kidney function improved. His blood pressure stabilised, and his doctor noted that his creatinine levels had decreased, indicating better kidney filtration. Mark also reported feeling more relaxed and energised, with less stress and anxiety in his daily life. He continued practising yoga as part of his routine and was able to manage his CKD with fewer medications.

This case highlights the effectiveness of yoga in supporting kidney health, especially in individuals looking for non-invasive, holistic approaches to managing kidney function and reducing stress.

Conclusion

Yoga offers a holistic approach to kidney health by improving circulation, reducing stress, and stimulating detoxification through targeted asanas and pranayama. Whether you are looking to maintain healthy kidney function or improve kidney health, yoga can be a powerful tool in your wellness routine. By incorporating gentle postures and mindful breathing exercises into your daily life, you can support your kidneys in their essential role of filtering waste and maintaining balance in the body.

Summary: Yoga for Kidney Health and Detoxification

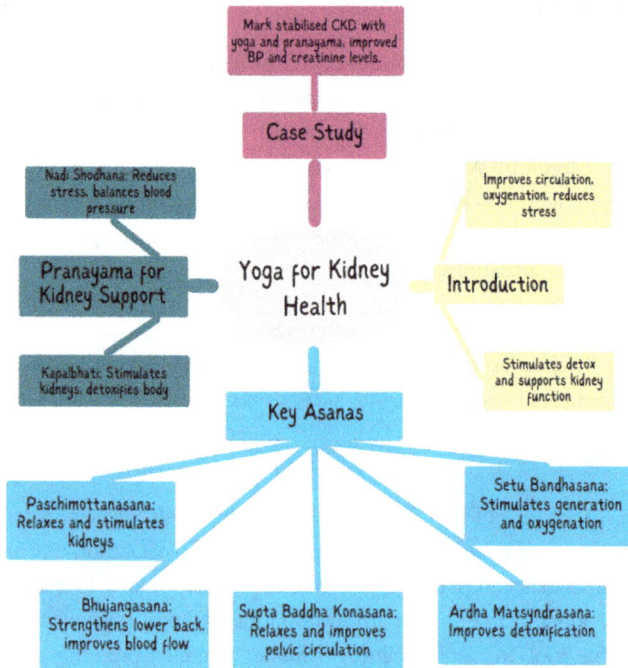

Mark stabilised CKD with yoga and pranayama, improved BP and creatinine levels.

Case Study

Nadi Shodhana: Reduces stress, balances blood pressure

Improves circulation, oxygenation, reduces stress

Pranayama for Kidney Support

Yoga for Kidney Health

Introduction

Kapalbhati: Stimulates kidneys, detoxifies body

Stimulates detox and supports kidney function

Key Asanas

Paschimottanasana: Relaxes and stimulates kidneys

Setu Bandhasana: Stimulates generation and oxygenation

Bhujangasana: Strengthens lower back, improves blood flow

Supta Baddha Konasana: Relaxes and improves pelvic circulation

Ardha Matsyndrasana: Improves detoxification

Chapter 5
Reflexology and Kidney Cleansing

Understanding Reflexology and Its Role in Kidney Health

Reflexology is a therapeutic practice based on the principle that specific points on the feet, hands, and ears correspond to different organs and systems in the body. By applying pressure to these reflex points, practitioners aim to stimulate the corresponding organs, promoting healing, improving circulation, and restoring balance. Reflexology has roots in ancient healing traditions from China, Egypt, and India, and today, it is widely used as a complementary therapy for a variety of health conditions, including kidney health.

The kidneys play a crucial role in detoxification, filtering waste products and excess fluids from the blood to form urine. Reflexology is believed to enhance this detoxification process by stimulating the reflex points associated with the kidneys, thereby improving blood flow, promoting the elimination of toxins, and supporting overall kidney function. Reflexology also induces relaxation, which can reduce stress—a significant contributor to kidney strain. Chronic stress raises cortisol levels, which can lead to high blood pressure, a major risk factor for kidney disease. Reflexology helps to lower cortisol and support healthier kidney function by calming the nervous system.

While reflexology is not a replacement for medical treatment, it can be a beneficial adjunct to therapies aimed at supporting kidney health, helping to balance the body's systems and promoting natural healing.

Key Reflex Points for the Kidneys on the Feet

In reflexology, the feet are mapped out to represent various organs, glands, and body systems. The kidney reflex points are located on the sole of each foot, specifically on the midline between the ball of the foot and the arch. Stimulating these points is thought to activate the kidneys and promote improved function.

Here's how to locate the kidney reflex points:

1. Right Kidney Reflex Point:

    a. On the sole of the right foot, find the area just below the ball of the foot, toward the centre of the arch. This point corresponds to the right kidney.

2. Left Kidney Reflex Point:

    a. Similarly, on the sole of the left foot, the reflex point for the left kidney is located just below the ball of the foot in the centre of the arch.

To activate the kidney reflex points, reflexologists apply firm yet gentle pressure, using techniques such as thumb walking or circular movements. Stimulating these points is believed to enhance the kidneys' ability to filter toxins and regulate fluid balance, helping to maintain optimal kidney function.

Additionally, there are other reflex points on the feet that influence the urinary system:

- **Bladder reflex points** are located just below the kidney points and can be stimulated to support the elimination of waste through urine.

- **Ureter reflex points** run from the kidney reflex points toward the bladder reflex points, representing the tubes that carry urine from the kidneys to the bladder.

Together, stimulating these points encourages a healthy flow of fluids and supports detoxification.

How Reflexology Supports Kidney Detoxification and Fluid Balance

Reflexology promotes kidney health in several ways, helping the kidneys to perform their essential functions of detoxification and fluid regulation:

1. **Improved Circulation to the Kidneys:** Reflexology stimulates blood flow to the kidneys, enhancing their ability to filter out toxins and waste products from the blood. This is particularly important for individuals with compromised kidney function, where circulation may be impaired. By increasing blood flow, reflexology helps the kidneys work more efficiently, supporting overall detoxification.

2. **Balancing Fluid Levels:** The kidneys are responsible for regulating the body's fluid balance, ensuring that the right amount of water and electrolytes are retained while excess fluids are excreted as urine. Reflexology can help improve the kidneys' ability to maintain this balance, preventing issues like water retention or dehydration. This is particularly beneficial for individuals dealing with swelling or oedema, conditions often linked to kidney dysfunction.

3. **Reducing Stress on the Kidneys:** Chronic stress can negatively impact kidney function, as elevated levels of cortisol and adrenaline increase blood pressure, placing a strain on the kidneys. Reflexology helps alleviate stress by inducing a deep state of relaxation, calming the nervous system, and lowering cortisol levels. This stress reduction helps protect the kidneys from damage caused by prolonged high blood pressure.

4. **Supporting Detox Pathways:** By stimulating the kidney reflex points and related areas on the feet, reflexology supports the body's natural detoxification pathways. As the kidneys are activated, they can more effectively filter out waste products like urea, creatinine, and excess salts from the bloodstream.

Reflexology can be beneficial during detox programs, where the kidneys play a crucial role in eliminating accumulated toxins.

5. **Promoting Relaxation and Pain Relief:** Reflexology is often used as a complementary therapy to relieve pain and discomfort. For individuals experiencing kidney-related pain, such as the discomfort associated with kidney stones or urinary tract infections, reflexology may provide relief by relaxing tense muscles, improving circulation, and reducing inflammation.

Case Study: Reflexology for Kidney Health in a 70-Year-Old Woman

Background: Margaret, a 70-year-old woman, had been managing high blood pressure for over a decade, which put her at risk for chronic kidney disease (CKD). During a routine check-up, her doctor noticed that her kidney function was beginning to decline, as indicated by elevated creatinine levels and a lower-than-normal glomerular filtration rate (GFR). Concerned about her kidney health, Margaret sought out complementary therapies to support her kidneys alongside her conventional medical treatment. Reflexology was recommended to help promote relaxation and stimulate kidney function.

Intervention: Margaret began receiving reflexology sessions twice a week from a certified reflexologist. Each session focused on stimulating the kidney reflex points on both feet, as well as the bladder and ureter points. The therapist used a combination of thumb walking and circular pressure techniques to activate these points. In addition to targeting the reflex points for the kidneys, the therapist also focused on general relaxation techniques to reduce Margaret's stress levels, which were contributing to her high blood pressure.

To support the therapy, Margaret was advised to increase her water intake, maintain a balanced diet with low sodium, and practice deep breathing exercises to reduce stress.

Outcome: After two months of regular reflexology sessions, Margaret experienced noticeable improvements in her overall well-being. Her blood pressure became more stable, and her doctor noted that her kidney function had stopped declining. While her creatinine levels remained higher than average, they did not worsen, and her GFR stabilised. Margaret also reported feeling more relaxed, with less tension in her body, and she found the sessions to be an essential part of her overall wellness routine.

Margaret's case highlights how reflexology can be a valuable complementary therapy for individuals with declining kidney function, particularly those who are looking to support their health naturally. Although reflexology did not reverse her kidney condition, it helped maintain her kidney function and improved her quality of life.

Conclusion

Reflexology offers a gentle, non-invasive way to support kidney health by stimulating key reflex points on the feet. Through improved circulation, enhanced detoxification, and stress reduction, reflexology helps the kidneys perform their vital functions more efficiently. Whether used as a preventive measure or as part of a holistic approach to managing kidney issues, reflexology can play an essential role in maintaining fluid balance, promoting relaxation, and supporting overall detoxification. By incorporating reflexology into your wellness routine, you can help protect and support your kidneys naturally.

Summary: Reflexology and Kidney Cleansing

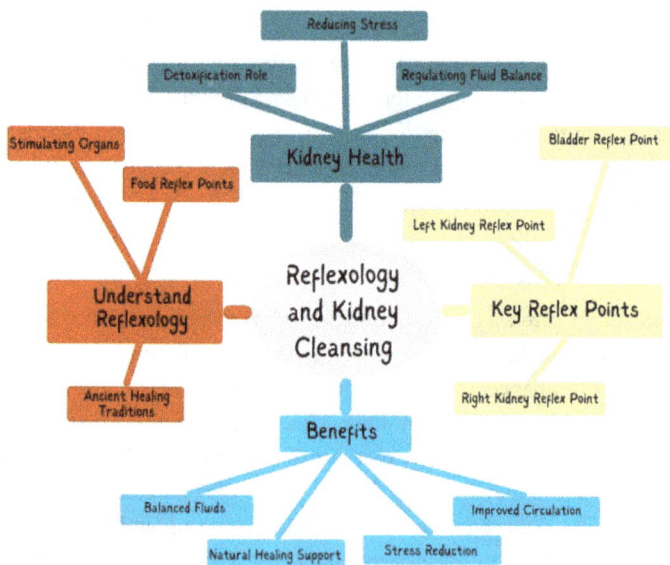

Reducing Stress

Detoxification Role

Regulating Fluid Balance

Kidney Health

Stimulating Organs

Food Reflex Points

Bladder Reflex Point

Left Kidney Reflex Point

Understand Reflexology

Reflexology and Kidney Cleansing

Key Reflex Points

Ancient Healing Traditions

Right Kidney Reflex Point

Benefits

Balanced Fluids

Improved Circulation

Natural Healing Support

Stress Reduction

Chapter 6
Acupuncture for Kidney Health

The Basics of Acupuncture and Its Role in Traditional Chinese Medicine (TCM)

Acupuncture is an ancient healing practice that has been a central component of Traditional Chinese Medicine (TCM) for thousands of years. It involves inserting thin, sterile needles into specific points on the body to balance energy flow, or **Qi** (pronounced "chee"). According to TCM, Qi flows through channels called **meridians**, which correspond to different organs and systems in the body. When Qi becomes blocked or imbalanced, illness or dysfunction can occur, affecting the health of the organs, including the kidneys.

Acupuncture helps restore the flow of Qi, promoting healing and improving the function of affected organs. It works by stimulating the body's natural ability to heal itself, encouraging blood flow, reducing inflammation, and modulating the nervous system. In the case of the kidneys, acupuncture is used to improve filtration function, reduce stress, and support detoxification.

Scientific studies have shown that acupuncture may also promote the release of endorphins and other neurotransmitters that help alleviate pain, reduce inflammation, and regulate blood pressure—all of which are important for maintaining kidney health. Acupuncture is particularly effective when used as part of a comprehensive approach to health, addressing not only physical symptoms but also the underlying energetic imbalances that contribute to disease.

Kidney Meridians and Key Acupuncture Points for Detoxification

In TCM, the kidneys are seen as the root of life and longevity, responsible for storing the body's vital essence (**Jing**) and governing growth, reproduction, and ageing. The **Kidney meridian** is one of the primary pathways that acupuncture practitioners focus on to support kidney function and detoxification. This meridian runs along the inside of the leg, starting from the sole of the foot and ascending to the chest. It contains several key acupuncture points that help balance and strengthen kidney energy, improve detoxification, and restore harmony to the body.

Here are some of the most important acupuncture points used to support kidney health:

1. Kidney 1 (K1) – Yongquan (Gushing Spring):

    a. **Location:** On the sole of the foot, about one-third of the distance between the toes and heel.

    b. **Function:** K1 is considered the most grounding acupuncture point, drawing energy down to calm the mind and reduce stress. It is used to treat symptoms of kidney deficiency, such as dizziness, tinnitus, and insomnia. Stimulating this point can also help regulate the kidneys' detoxification processes and improve fluid balance.

2. Kidney 3 (K3) – Taixi (Supreme Stream):

    a. **Location:** Just behind the inner ankle bone, in the depression between the ankle and the Achilles tendon.

    b. **Function:** K3 is one of the most powerful points for tonifying the kidneys. It is used to boost kidney energy (Qi), support kidney function, and promote detoxification. It is often recommended for symptoms of fatigue, lower back pain, and frequent urination, all of which are linked to kidney imbalances.

3. Kidney 7 (K7) – Fuliu (Returning Current):

    a. **Location:** Approximately two fingers' width above the inner ankle bone, along the Kidney meridian.

    b. **Function:** K7 is a key point for regulating water metabolism and supporting the kidneys in maintaining fluid balance. It is commonly used in cases of oedema, night sweats, or difficulty urinating, as well as for enhancing the kidneys' ability to filter toxins.

4. Bladder 23 (B23) – Shenshu (Kidney Shu):

    a. **Location:** On the lower back, 1.5 inches lateral to the second lumbar vertebra.

    b. **Function:** Although part of the **Bladder meridian,** B23 is a vital point for kidney health, as it directly influences the kidneys and adrenal glands. Stimulating this point helps strengthen the kidneys, improve circulation to the area, and reduce lower back pain often associated with kidney imbalances.

These acupuncture points, when stimulated, activate the flow of Qi through the Kidney meridian and support the kidneys' role in filtering blood, eliminating waste, and maintaining overall balance in the body. By harmonising the flow of Qi along this meridian, acupuncture helps the kidneys perform their detoxification functions more efficiently.

How Acupuncture Balances Yin and Yang in the Kidneys

In TCM, the concept of **Yin** and **Yang** is fundamental to understanding how the body maintains balance and health. Yin represents the cooling, nourishing, and restorative aspects of the body, while Yang embodies warmth, activity, and energy. The kidneys are considered the source of both Yin and Yang energy in the body, and maintaining a balance between these two forces is essential for optimal kidney function.

When there is a deficiency of **Kidney Yin**, the body may experience symptoms such as:

- Dryness, including dry mouth and skin
- Hot flashes or night sweats
- Dizziness and tinnitus
- Low back pain or weakness

When there is a deficiency of **Kidney Yang**, symptoms can include:

- Cold hands and feet
- Fatigue and lethargy
- Water retention or oedema
- Frequent urination, especially at night

Acupuncture works to balance the Yin and Yang energies in the kidneys by targeting specific points along the Kidney meridian. For instance, stimulating **K3** and **B23** can tonify Kidney Yang, warming the body and improving circulation. On the other hand, stimulating **K1** and **K7** can nourish Kidney Yin, helping to cool the body and restore fluid balance.

By balancing Yin and Yang in the kidneys, acupuncture supports the body's natural detoxification processes, boosts energy levels, and helps maintain overall health. This balancing act is crucial for preventing kidney imbalances that can lead to conditions such as chronic kidney disease, high blood pressure, or urinary issues.

Case Study: Acupuncture to Support Kidney Function in a 50-Year-Old Client

Background: David, a 50-year-old man, was experiencing early signs of kidney dysfunction. His doctor noted elevated creatinine levels and early-stage hypertension, which put him at risk for chronic kidney disease (CKD). David also reported frequent urination at night, fatigue, and lower back pain, all of which are common symptoms of kidney deficiency in TCM. Concerned about his kidney health, David sought out acupuncture as a complementary therapy to improve his kidney function and overall well-being.

Intervention: David began receiving acupuncture treatments once a week from a licensed acupuncturist. The acupuncturist focused on key kidney points, including **K3**, **K7**, and **B23**, to strengthen Kidney Qi, regulate water metabolism, and address his back pain. Additionally, the practitioner used **K1** to reduce stress and calm David's nervous system, helping lower his blood pressure.

In conjunction with acupuncture, David was advised to adopt simple lifestyle changes, including staying hydrated, reducing his intake of salty and processed foods, and practising mindfulness exercises to manage stress.

Outcome: After six weeks of acupuncture treatments, David reported significant improvements. His creatinine levels stabilised, and his doctor noted a slight reduction in his blood pressure. David also experienced fewer episodes of nighttime urination and had more energy throughout the day. His lower back pain diminished, and he felt more balanced and relaxed overall. The combination of acupuncture and lifestyle changes supported his kidney health and prevented further decline in function.

David's case demonstrates how acupuncture can be an effective complementary therapy for individuals with early-stage kidney dysfunction, particularly when used alongside other health interventions. By balancing the body's energy and promoting detoxification, acupuncture helped David manage his symptoms and improve his overall kidney health.

Conclusion

Acupuncture offers a holistic approach to supporting kidney health by stimulating key meridian points, balancing Yin and Yang energies, and promoting detoxification. By improving circulation, reducing stress, and regulating fluid balance, acupuncture helps the kidneys function more efficiently, allowing them to perform their vital role in the body's detoxification system. Whether used as a preventive measure or as part of a comprehensive treatment plan, acupuncture can play an important role in maintaining kidney health and supporting long-term well-being.

Summary:

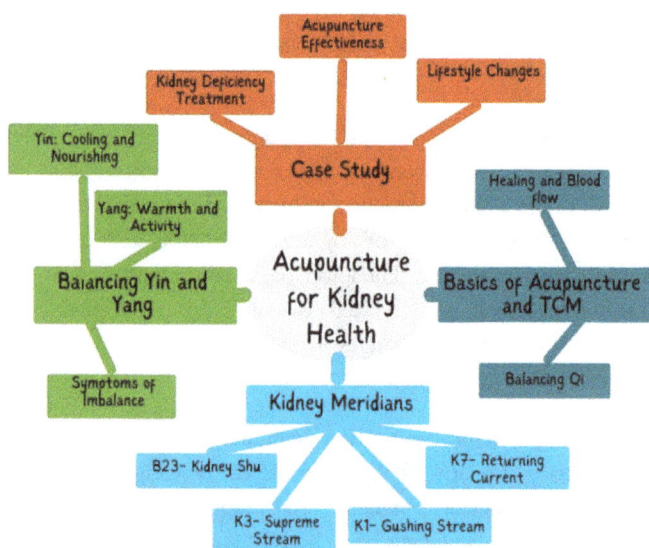

Chapter 7
Traditional Chinese Medicine (TCM) and Kidney Detox

The Importance of Kidney Health in TCM Philosophy

In Traditional Chinese Medicine (TCM), the kidneys are considered the foundation of life and vitality, responsible for governing the body's essential energy, known as **Qi**. The kidneys hold a unique place in TCM philosophy as the "storehouse" of both **Jing** (vital essence) and the **root of Yin and Yang**. This perspective highlights the kidneys not only as physical organs responsible for filtering waste but also as the root of the body's life force, vitality, and longevity.

The kidneys in TCM are believed to control growth, development, reproduction, and ageing, as well as being closely tied to the body's ability to detoxify and maintain balance. Kidney health, therefore, is not limited to preventing disease—it is about preserving life energy, promoting overall wellness, and maintaining long-term health.

When kidney energy (known as **Kidney Qi**) is strong, a person is considered to have robust health, physical strength, and vitality. However, when the kidneys become imbalanced—whether due to age, stress, overwork, or environmental factors—this can result in weakness, fatigue, and a range of physical and emotional symptoms, including lower back pain, dizziness, tinnitus, and even premature ageing.

TCM views the kidneys as not just organs of elimination but as the centre of the body's life force, playing a vital role in growth, reproduction, and the ability to resist disease. Therefore, maintaining kidney health is essential for overall detoxification, resilience, and longevity.

Key Herbs in TCM for Supporting Kidney Function

Herbal medicine is a cornerstone of TCM, and specific herbs have been used for thousands of years to support kidney health, strengthen Kidney Qi, and promote detoxification. Among the most important herbs in TCM for kidney health are **Rehmannia** and **Cordyceps**.

1. Rehmannia (Shu Di Huang)

    Rehmannia is one of the most important herbs in TCM for nourishing **Kidney Yin** and replenishing **Jing**. It is often used to treat conditions related to kidney deficiency, such as fatigue, dizziness, tinnitus, and lower back pain. Rehmannia helps to replenish the vital energy stored in the kidneys, making it particularly effective for individuals who are experiencing depletion due to stress, overwork, or ageing.

    a. **How it works:** Rehmannia helps to restore balance to the body by replenishing fluids, cooling excess heat, and nourishing the kidneys' Yin energy. It is often combined with other herbs to enhance its tonifying effects and is frequently used in formulas to treat symptoms associated with kidney Yin deficiency, such as dry mouth, hot flashes, and night sweats.

    b. **Common use:** Rehmannia is commonly used in formulas such as **Liu Wei Di Huang Wan** (Six Flavour Rehmannia Pill), which is widely prescribed for replenishing Kidney Yin and supporting overall vitality.

2. Cordyceps (Dong Chong Xia Cao)

    Cordyceps is a powerful medicinal fungus that is highly prized in TCM for its ability to tonify **Kidney Yang** and enhance energy, stamina, and vitality. It is often used to treat symptoms of kidney Yang deficiency, such as cold hands and feet, frequent urination, and fatigue. Cordyceps is also known for its immune-boosting properties and its ability to improve oxygen utilisation, making it a popular herb for enhancing athletic performance and recovery.

a. **How it works:** Cordyceps strengthens Kidney Yang, which is the warming, active energy that powers the body's functions. It helps improve circulation, supports the adrenal glands, and enhances the body's ability to handle stress. Cordyceps is also known for improving kidney function in individuals with chronic kidney disease, as it has been shown to reduce proteinuria (excess protein in the urine) and improve kidney filtration rates.

b. **Common use:** Cordyceps is used in many TCM formulas to boost energy, enhance lung function, and support kidney health. It is often combined with herbs like Rehmannia in formulas designed to balance both Kidney Yin and Yang.

Other important herbs for kidney health in TCM include **Astragalus (Huang Qi)** for strengthening Qi and enhancing immune function, and **He Shou Wu (Fo-Ti)**, which nourishes Kidney Yin and helps prevent the signs of ageing. Together, these herbs create a balanced approach to maintaining kidney health by addressing both the cooling and nourishing aspects of Kidney Yin and the warming, energising aspects of Kidney Yang.

The Concept of Qi and Kidney Essence (Jing)

In TCM, **Qi** is the vital energy that flows through the body, sustaining life and supporting every physiological function. The kidneys are considered the source of **Pre-Natal Qi**, which is the Qi that we are born with, inherited from our parents. This Pre-Natal Qi, also known as **Jing**, is a vital essence stored in the kidneys that determines our lifespan, vitality, and resistance to disease.

Jing is seen as the foundation of growth, reproduction, and ageing. When we are young, we have an abundant supply of Jing, which supports physical development, fertility, and vitality. However, as we age, our Jing becomes depleted, leading to the natural process of ageing, reduced energy levels, and increased susceptibility to illness.

Kidney health, therefore, is directly tied to the preservation of Jing. The better we care for our kidneys, the more we can conserve our Jing, slowing the ageing process and maintaining vitality well into old age. In TCM, this is why maintaining kidney health is seen as essential not just for detoxification but for overall longevity and well-being.

Practices such as **Qi Gong**, **Tai Chi**, and **meditation** are often recommended to help cultivate Qi and preserve Jing. In addition, certain herbal formulas, like those containing Rehmannia and Cordyceps, are prescribed to replenish and protect Kidney Jing, preventing premature ageing and promoting long-term health.

Balancing **Kidney Yin and Yang** is also crucial to maintaining the flow of Qi and the preservation of Jing. **Kidney Yin** represents the cooling, nourishing, and restorative energy, while **Kidney Yang** symbolises the warming, active, and energising forces. A balance between these two forces is essential for optimal kidney function, as an imbalance can lead to either depletion (Kidney Yin deficiency) or overactivity (Kidney Yang deficiency).

Case Study: Using TCM for Kidney Health in a 35-Year-Old Athlete

Background: Sarah, a 35-year-old competitive athlete, began experiencing symptoms of fatigue, lower back pain, and frequent urination after months of intense training for a triathlon. Despite being in excellent physical shape, Sarah felt that her energy levels were unusually low and that she was struggling to recover between workouts. After visiting a TCM practitioner, it was determined that Sarah was experiencing symptoms of **Kidney Yang deficiency**, likely due to the physical stress and overwork her body had endured during training.

Intervention: The TCM practitioner recommended a combination of acupuncture and herbal therapy to restore balance to Sarah's kidneys and support her recovery. Sarah was prescribed a formula containing **Cordyceps** and **Rehmannia**, designed to tonify both Kidney Yang and Kidney Yin. Cordyceps was included to enhance her stamina and improve her recovery time. At the same time, Rehmannia helped nourish her depleted Kidney Yin and restore fluid balance.

In addition to the herbal treatment, Sarah underwent weekly acupuncture sessions to strengthen Kidney Qi and balance her energy flow. The acupuncture focused on key points along the Kidney meridian, such as **K3** and **B23**, to improve energy levels, reduce fatigue, and alleviate her lower back pain.

Outcome: After six weeks of treatment, Sarah's symptoms began to improve. Her energy levels increased, and she found that she was able to recover more quickly from her workouts. The lower back pain and frequent urination also subsided. Her TCM practitioner continued to adjust her herbal formula throughout the course of her training, ensuring that both Kidney Yin and Yang were balanced. By the end of her treatment, Sarah felt more energised and resilient, and she was able to complete her triathlon without any further issues.

This case illustrates how TCM can be used to support kidney health in athletes or individuals undergoing physical stress. By balancing Kidney Yin and Yang and replenishing vital energy stores with herbs like Cordyceps and Rehmannia, Sarah was able to enhance her athletic performance, recover from physical strain, and protect her kidneys from long-term damage.

Conclusion

Traditional Chinese Medicine offers a unique and holistic approach to kidney health, emphasising the importance of balancing Kidney Qi, preserving Jing, and supporting both Kidney Yin and Yang. By using powerful herbs like Rehmannia and Cordyceps, TCM provides a natural way to strengthen kidney function, enhance detoxification, and promote longevity. Whether you are dealing with physical stress, ageing, or chronic kidney issues, TCM's focus on kidney health can help you maintain vitality and well-being throughout your life.

Summary: Traditional Chinese Medicine (TCM) and Kidney Detox

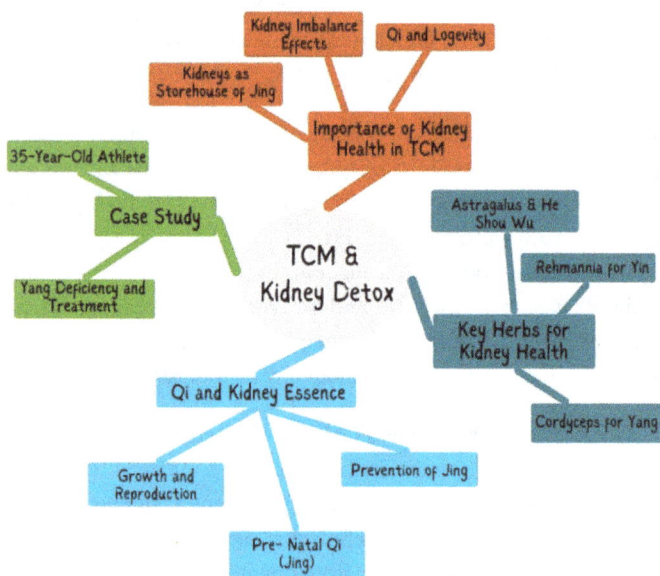

Chapter 8
Ayurveda and Kidney Cleansing

The Ayurvedic Approach to Kidney Health and the Dosha System

Ayurveda, the ancient system of medicine that originated in India over 5,000 years ago, views the body as a balance of three energies or **doshas—Vata**, **Pitta**, and **Kapha**. Each dosha represents different physiological functions and traits. In Ayurvedic philosophy, maintaining balance among these doshas is essential for good health. The kidneys are considered vital organs that help regulate the body's fluid balance, cleanse toxins (known as **Ama** in Ayurveda), and support overall health.

In Ayurveda, kidney health is linked to the balance of **Kapha** and **Vata** doshas. Kapha governs structure and fluid balance in the body, including water retention and kidney function. An imbalance in Kapha can lead to conditions like water retention, kidney stones, or slow metabolism. On the other hand, **Vata** governs movement, including the flow of urine and the elimination of waste. When Vata is out of balance, it can cause dehydration, excessive urination, or dry tissues, which can negatively impact kidney function.

Ayurveda emphasises the importance of keeping the body's detoxification systems in optimal condition to prevent the accumulation of Ama (toxins), which can block energy channels and impair kidney function. Ayurvedic practitioners recommend maintaining a lifestyle and diet that balances the doshas, promotes digestion, and supports the natural detoxification processes of the kidneys.

Key Ayurvedic Herbs for Kidney Cleansing

Ayurveda utilises a wide range of herbs that are known to support kidney health and promote detoxification. Two of the most important herbs for kidney cleansing are **Punarnava** and **Gokshura**.

1.   Punarnava (Boerhavia diffusa):

Punarnava, whose name means "one that renews or rejuvenates the body," is a powerful herb used in Ayurveda to support kidney function and cleanse excess water and toxins. It has diuretic properties, which help to promote the flow of urine and prevent water retention. Punarnava is also an anti-inflammatory herb that helps protect kidney tissue from damage and reduce swelling or oedema caused by kidney dysfunction.

   a.   **How it works:** Punarnava supports the kidneys by promoting the elimination of fluids and toxins through the urine. It enhances kidney function by reducing inflammation and protecting the renal system from oxidative stress. Punarnava is often recommended for individuals dealing with water retention, urinary tract infections, or early-stage kidney disease.

   b.   **Common use:** Punarnava is often used in Ayurvedic formulas designed to treat kidney issues, fluid retention, and urinary health. It is available as a powdered herb, tincture, or in herbal capsules.

2.   Gokshura (Tribulus terrestris):

Gokshura is a well-known Ayurvedic herb used to support kidney health, urinary tract function, and overall detoxification. It acts as a natural diuretic, helping to clear toxins from the kidneys while preventing the formation of kidney stones. Gokshura is also considered a rejuvenating herb that strengthens the kidneys and improves their filtration function.

a. **How it works:** Gokshura supports the kidneys by promoting the natural flow of urine and reducing the risk of kidney stones. Its anti-inflammatory and antioxidant properties help protect the kidneys from oxidative damage, making it beneficial for people with compromised kidney function. Additionally, Gokshura is believed to improve overall vitality and energy, which are closely connected to kidney health in Ayurveda.

b. **Common use:** Gokshura is commonly taken as part of an Ayurvedic formulation for kidney health, either in powder form, tincture, or herbal supplements. It is also used in formulas aimed at promoting urinary health and preventing stone formation.

Both Punarnava and Gokshura are considered **Rasayanas** in Ayurveda—herbs that rejuvenate and restore balance to the body's systems. They work synergistically to improve kidney function, promote detoxification, and balance fluid levels in the body.

Panchakarma: Ayurvedic Detoxification Practices for Kidney Support

Panchakarma is Ayurveda's signature detoxification therapy, designed to cleanse the body of toxins, balance the doshas, and rejuvenate the organs, including the kidneys. Panchakarma consists of five purification techniques that remove accumulated toxins (Ama) from the body, improving overall health and restoring balance. These techniques are customised based on an individual's dosha constitution and current health condition, making Panchakarma a deeply personalised detoxification experience.

For kidney health, Panchakarma focuses on clearing excess **Kapha** (fluid and mucus) and balancing **Vata** (responsible for elimination and movement). The following Panchakarma practices are particularly beneficial for supporting kidney function and detoxification:

1. Virechana (Therapeutic Purgation):

Virechana is a controlled cleansing process that involves the use of herbal laxatives to eliminate toxins from the liver and kidneys via the digestive system. This practice helps clear the body of excess Pitta (heat and toxins), which can overwhelm the kidneys. By improving liver function and reducing Pitta, Virechana helps the kidneys work more efficiently, supporting detoxification.

2. Basti (Herbal Enema):

Basti is considered one of the most important detox therapies in Ayurveda, particularly for balancing Vata. It involves the administration of herbal oil or decoctions through the colon to cleanse the lower digestive tract and remove toxins. Basti helps nourish and rejuvenate the kidneys by improving elimination and preventing constipation, which can aggravate kidney function. It is especially effective for those experiencing kidney issues related to Vata imbalance, such as dehydration and excessive urination.

3. Abhyanga (Oil Massage):

Abhyanga is an Ayurvedic oil massage that uses warm, medicated oils to stimulate circulation, promote detoxification, and nourish the tissues. For kidney health, Abhyanga helps improve lymphatic drainage, reduce water retention, and relax the body, making it easier for the kidneys to eliminate toxins. The practice also calms the nervous system, reducing stress—a key factor in maintaining kidney function.

4. Swedana (Herbal Steam Therapy):

Swedana involves herbal steam therapy to open the pores and encourage the release of toxins through sweat. This practice enhances kidney function by improving circulation and supporting the body's natural detoxification pathways. Swedana helps reduce water retention and promotes the removal of toxins from the skin, taking some of the burden off the kidneys.

By undergoing Panchakarma, individuals can remove accumulated toxins that impair kidney function and rebalance their doshas, leading to improved kidney health and overall vitality.

Case Study: A 45-Year-Old Woman's Journey to Kidney Health through Ayurveda

Background: Maria, a 45-year-old woman, had been experiencing symptoms of fluid retention, frequent urination, and lower back pain. After a series of tests, her doctor diagnosed her with early-stage kidney dysfunction, likely linked to stress and dehydration. Looking for a natural approach to support her kidneys, Maria decided to explore Ayurvedic treatment, seeking help from an Ayurvedic practitioner.

Intervention: The Ayurvedic practitioner assessed Maria's condition and identified an imbalance in **Kapha** and **Vata** doshas, contributing to her symptoms. The practitioner recommended a personalised treatment plan that included herbal therapy, diet modifications, and Panchakarma.

Maria was prescribed **Punarnava** to reduce water retention and inflammation and **Gokshura** to strengthen her kidney function and improve filtration. In addition to these herbs, she underwent a **Panchakarma** cleanse, which included **Basti** (herbal enema) to balance Vata and **Abhyanga** (oil massage) to reduce stress and promote circulation.

Maria was also advised to follow a Kapha-reducing diet, which included light, warm, and easily digestible foods, along with increased hydration to support kidney function. She was encouraged to practise gentle yoga and meditation to reduce stress and improve overall vitality.

Outcome: After two months of Ayurvedic treatment, Maria noticed significant improvements. Her fluid retention decreased, and she no longer experienced frequent urination. Her lower back pain also subsided, and she felt more energised. Follow-up tests showed that her kidney function had stabilised, with no further decline. The combination of herbal therapy, Panchakarma, and lifestyle changes helped Maria restore balance to her body and support her kidneys' natural detoxification processes.

Maria's case highlights the effectiveness of Ayurveda in addressing kidney imbalances through personalised treatments that target the root cause of dysfunction. By balancing her doshas and using specific kidney-cleansing herbs, Maria was able to improve her kidney function and enhance her overall well-being.

Conclusion

Ayurveda provides a comprehensive approach to kidney health, emphasising the importance of balancing the doshas, promoting detoxification, and using natural herbs to support kidney function. Through the use of powerful herbs like Punarnava and Gokshura, along with detoxification practices like Panchakarma, Ayurveda offers a holistic way to cleanse the kidneys, prevent disease, and maintain overall vitality. Whether you are dealing with early-stage kidney dysfunction or simply seeking to enhance your kidney health, Ayurveda provides effective, time-tested strategies for maintaining balance and well-being.

Summary:

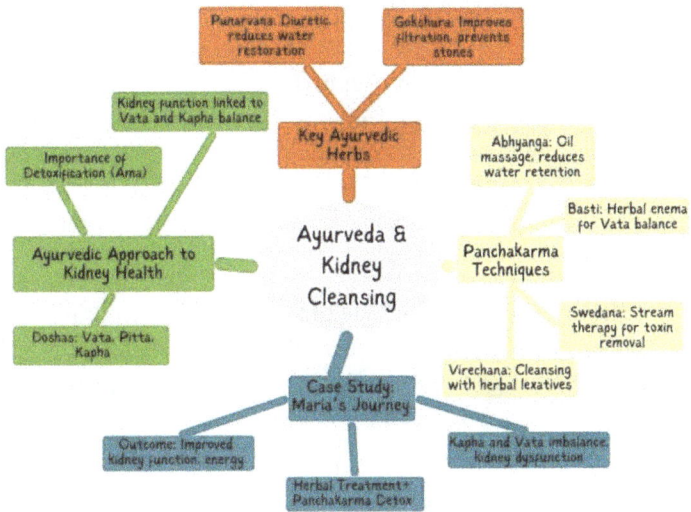

Chapter 9
Diet and Hydration for Kidney Health

The Role of Proper Hydration in Kidney Detoxification

Water is essential for every organ in the body, and for the kidneys, proper hydration is critical for optimal function and detoxification. The kidneys' primary role is to filter blood, remove waste products, and balance fluids. Without enough water, the kidneys struggle to perform these vital tasks, leading to an accumulation of toxins and impaired kidney function.

When the body is well-hydrated, blood flows more freely through the kidneys, allowing them to efficiently filter out toxins and waste products, such as urea and creatinine, while maintaining electrolyte balance. Inadequate hydration, on the other hand, can lead to concentrated urine, which increases the risk of kidney stones, urinary tract infections, and other complications.

Dehydration also causes stress on the kidneys, as they have to work harder to retain fluids and concentrate waste in the urine. This can lead to kidney damage over time, making it important to ensure that you drink enough water throughout the day to support kidney health. The general recommendation is to drink at least **8 cups (2 litres)** of water daily, but individual needs may vary based on factors like age, activity level, and climate.

For those with kidney disease or compromised kidney function, it is important to discuss your hydration needs with a healthcare provider, as fluid intake may need to be adjusted. While hydration is essential for kidney health, excessive water intake can place undue strain on already weakened kidneys. Thus, balance is key.

Foods that Support Kidney Health

In addition to proper hydration, a healthy diet plays a crucial role in maintaining kidney function and promoting detoxification. Certain foods are particularly beneficial for the kidneys due to their high levels of antioxidants, vitamins, and minerals. These foods help reduce oxidative stress, support detox pathways, and prevent inflammation, which can harm the kidneys. Three kidney-supportive foods include **beets**, **blueberries**, and **cabbage**.

1. Beets

    Beets are rich in nitrates, which help improve blood flow and reduce blood pressure—key factors in maintaining healthy kidney function. The nitrates in beets help dilate blood vessels, making it easier for blood to flow through the kidneys and filter out waste products. Beets are also high in antioxidants, such as betalains, which help reduce inflammation and oxidative stress in the kidneys.

    a. How to include beets in your diet:

    b. Beets can be eaten raw in salads, roasted as a side dish, or blended into smoothies. Beet juice is also a convenient way to support kidney health, but it is important to choose fresh, unsweetened varieties.

2. Blueberries

    Blueberries are packed with antioxidants, particularly **anthocyanins**, which protect the kidneys from damage caused by oxidative stress and inflammation. Blueberries also help lower blood pressure and improve heart health, both of which are essential for supporting kidney function. Their low potassium content makes them a kidney-friendly fruit, especially for those with chronic kidney disease (CKD), who may need to limit potassium intake.

    a. How to include blueberries in your diet:

Blueberries can be eaten fresh, frozen, or added to oatmeal, yoghurt, or smoothies. They make a great snack and are an excellent choice for those looking to support kidney health while enjoying a low-sugar, nutrient-dense fruit.

3.   Cabbage

Cabbage is a cruciferous vegetable that is low in potassium and packed with vitamins C and K, fibre, and phytochemicals that protect against oxidative stress and inflammation. Cabbage contains compounds called **glucosinolates**, which help detoxify the kidneys by neutralising toxins and supporting liver function. Cabbage is also rich in fibre, which aids digestion and prevents the buildup of waste products that can strain the kidneys.

a.   How to include cabbage in your diet:

Cabbage can be eaten raw in salads, fermented into sauerkraut for added probiotic benefits, or cooked as a side dish. Its versatility makes it an excellent addition to any kidney-friendly diet.

Nutritional Tips for Maintaining Kidney Health

Maintaining kidney health requires more than just eating specific foods—it also involves adopting dietary habits that promote overall wellness and reduce strain on the kidneys. Here are some key nutritional tips to keep your kidneys healthy:

1.   Limit Sodium Intake:

Excessive sodium can lead to high blood pressure, which places strain on the kidneys and increases the risk of kidney damage. Aim to consume no more than **2,300 milligrams of sodium per day**, and avoid processed and packaged foods, which are often high in hidden sodium. Instead, season your meals with herbs and spices to add flavour without the added salt.

2.   Reduce Protein Overload:

While protein is essential for health, consuming too much protein—especially from animal sources—can burden the kidneys, as they must work harder to eliminate the waste products of protein metabolism. For those with healthy kidneys, it is important to maintain a balanced intake of protein, but for individuals with compromised kidney function, reducing protein intake may help slow the progression of kidney disease. Plant-based protein sources, such as beans, lentils, and tofu, are often gentler on the kidneys.

3.   Limit Processed Foods:

Processed foods are often high in sodium, phosphorus, and unhealthy fats, all of which can negatively impact kidney function. Instead of reaching for processed snacks, opt for whole, unprocessed foods like fruits, vegetables, and whole grains, which provide essential nutrients without the harmful additives.

4.   Stay Hydrated with Water-Rich Foods:

In addition to drinking water, eating water-rich foods, such as cucumbers, melons, and leafy greens, can help keep the body hydrated and support kidney function. These foods also provide essential vitamins and minerals that help maintain electrolyte balance.

5.   Monitor Potassium and Phosphorus Intake (for CKD Patients):

For individuals with chronic kidney disease (CKD), it is important to monitor potassium and phosphorus intake, as the kidneys may struggle to eliminate excess amounts of these minerals. Foods like bananas, potatoes, dairy products, and nuts are high in potassium and phosphorus, and may need to be limited or replaced with lower-potassium and phosphorus alternatives, such as apples, cauliflower, and rice.

6.   Incorporate Anti-Inflammatory Foods:

Chronic inflammation can damage the kidneys over time. Incorporating anti-inflammatory foods like turmeric, ginger, garlic, and leafy greens into your diet can help reduce inflammation and protect kidney function. These foods are also rich in antioxidants, which neutralise free radicals and reduce oxidative stress on the kidneys.

By following these nutritional guidelines and focusing on a balanced, kidney-friendly diet, you can support the health of your kidneys and reduce the risk of developing kidney-related issues over time.

Case Study: A 25-Year-Old Athlete Improves Kidney Health with a Simple Diet Shift

Background: David, a 25-year-old competitive swimmer, had been experiencing frequent muscle cramps, fatigue, and dark-coloured urine after intense training sessions. Concerned about his hydration levels and overall kidney health, he consulted a nutritionist who recommended a few dietary changes to support his kidneys and improve his recovery.

Intervention: David's nutritionist explained that his high-protein, low-carbohydrate diet—while beneficial for muscle building—was putting strain on his kidneys, as they were working overtime to process excess protein and eliminate waste products. The nutritionist recommended that David reduce his intake of animal protein and incorporate more plant-based protein sources, such as lentils, quinoa, and tofu, into his meals.

Additionally, David was advised to increase his water intake and include more water-rich foods in his diet, such as cucumbers, watermelon, and leafy greens. To support kidney detoxification, his nutritionist also suggested that he incorporate beets and blueberries into his daily meals for their antioxidant and anti-inflammatory benefits.

Outcome: After following the diet recommendations for six weeks, David noticed a significant improvement in his energy levels, hydration status, and overall kidney function. His muscle cramps diminished, and his urine returned to a healthy, pale yellow colour—indicating improved hydration. David also reported faster recovery after training sessions and less overall fatigue. His simple dietary adjustments not only supported his athletic performance but also improved his kidney health and reduced strain on his kidneys.

This case highlights how simple dietary changes—such as reducing excess protein, increasing hydration, and incorporating kidney-friendly foods—can have a profound impact on kidney health, even for young and active individuals.

Conclusion

Diet and hydration are fundamental to maintaining healthy kidneys and supporting the body's natural detoxification processes. By consuming the right foods—such as beets, blueberries, and cabbage—and staying well-hydrated, you can help your kidneys filter out toxins, balance fluids, and reduce the risk of kidney damage. Whether you are an athlete or simply someone looking to improve your overall health, adopting a kidney-friendly diet is an effective way to support long-term kidney function and well-being.

Summary:

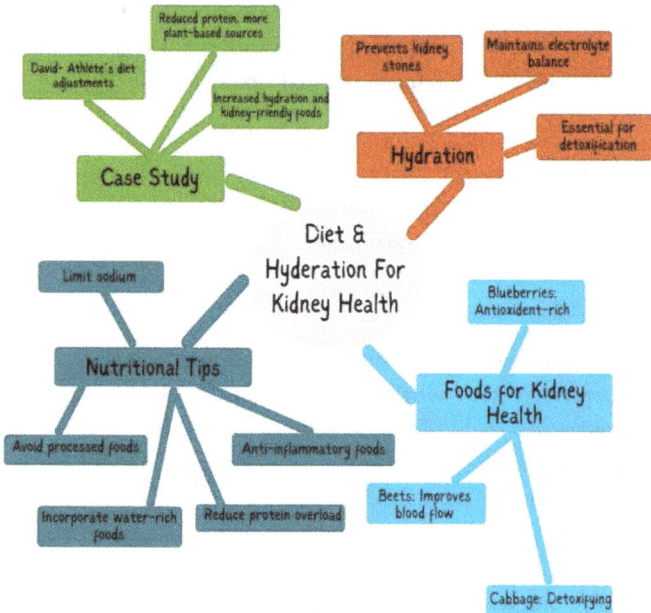

Diet & Hydration For Kidney Health

Case Study
- David- Athlete's diet adjustments
- Reduced protein, more plant-based sources
- Increased hydration and kidney-friendly foods

Hydration
- Prevents kidney stones
- Maintains electrolyte balance
- Essential for detoxification

Nutritional Tips
- Limit sodium
- Avoid processed foods
- Anti-inflammatory foods
- Incorporate water-rich foods
- Reduce protein overload

Foods for Kidney Health
- Blueberries: Antioxident-rich
- Beets: Improves blood flow
- Cabbage: Detoxifying

Chapter 10
Herbal Supplements and Phytochemicals for Kidney Detox

Top Herbs and Nutraceuticals for Kidney Health

Herbal supplements and phytochemicals have long been used in traditional medicine systems like Ayurveda and Traditional Chinese Medicine to support kidney health and enhance the body's natural detoxification processes. These natural remedies work by promoting kidney function, improving circulation, and reducing inflammation in the renal system. While diet and hydration are critical for kidney health, certain herbs and nutraceuticals provide additional support, especially for those experiencing mild kidney stress or looking to maintain optimal kidney function. Three key herbs and nutraceuticals for kidney health include **dandelion**, **nettle**, and **N-acetyl cysteine (NAC)**.

1. Dandelion (Taraxacum officinale)

    Dandelion is a potent diuretic and kidney tonic that has been used for centuries to support kidney and liver health. Known for its ability to promote urine production and reduce water retention, dandelion helps the kidneys eliminate waste products more effectively. It is particularly beneficial for individuals experiencing fluid retention, high blood pressure, or mild kidney inflammation.

    a. **How it works:** Dandelion supports kidney detoxification by increasing urine output, which helps flush out toxins and reduce the buildup of waste products in the blood. It also contains antioxidants that protect kidney cells from oxidative stress. Additionally, dandelion's high potassium content helps balance electrolytes, making it a suitable herb for supporting kidney health in a balanced way.

b. **Common use:** Dandelion can be consumed as a tea, tincture, or capsule. Many herbal formulations for kidney detoxification include dandelion as a key ingredient due to its diuretic and cleansing properties.

2. Nettle (Urtica dioica)

Nettle is another powerful herb used to support kidney function and promote detoxification. Known for its diuretic properties, nettle helps increase urine flow, which aids in the elimination of toxins and excess fluids from the body. Nettle is also rich in vitamins and minerals, such as iron and calcium, which support kidney health and overall vitality.

a. **How it works:** Nettle helps reduce inflammation in the kidneys, making it an excellent choice for individuals dealing with chronic kidney inflammation or urinary tract issues. Its diuretic properties support fluid balance and reduce the risk of kidney stones by encouraging the elimination of minerals that could form stones. Nettle also acts as an anti-inflammatory, protecting kidney tissues from damage caused by chronic conditions such as diabetes or hypertension.

b. **Common use:** Nettle is commonly consumed as an herbal tea or in capsule form. It can also be taken as a tincture for individuals looking for a concentrated dose of its kidney-supporting properties.

3. N-acetyl cysteine (NAC)

NAC is a precursor to **glutathione**, the body's most powerful antioxidant, and plays a crucial role in protecting the kidneys from oxidative stress. NAC supports kidney health by replenishing glutathione levels, reducing inflammation, and protecting the kidneys from the damaging effects of toxins and medications. It is particularly beneficial for individuals at risk of kidney damage due to conditions like diabetes, high blood pressure, or frequent use of nephrotoxic medications.

a. **How it works:** NAC helps neutralise free radicals and reduces oxidative stress in the kidneys, preventing cellular damage that can lead to chronic kidney disease. It also supports detoxification pathways in the liver, which indirectly benefits the kidneys by reducing the overall toxic load on the body.

b. **Common use:** NAC is available in capsule or powder form and is often taken as a daily supplement to support kidney health and enhance detoxification processes.

In addition to these herbs and nutraceuticals, others such as **turmeric** (for its anti-inflammatory properties) and **ginger** (for improving circulation) also provide benefits to kidney health. When used appropriately, these supplements can offer a natural way to enhance kidney detoxification and support long-term kidney function.

What to Avoid: Nephrotoxic (Kidney-Damaging) Substances

While certain herbs and supplements can promote kidney health, it is equally important to avoid substances that can cause harm to the kidneys. **Nephrotoxic substances** are those that can damage kidney tissue, impair kidney function, or contribute to the development of kidney disease. Here are some of the most common nephrotoxic substances to avoid:

1. Non-Steroidal Anti-Inflammatory Drugs (NSAIDs):

Medications like ibuprofen and naproxen are commonly used to reduce pain and inflammation, but regular or excessive use can strain the kidneys. NSAIDs reduce blood flow to the kidneys, which can impair their ability to filter waste and lead to kidney damage over time. Individuals with pre-existing kidney conditions or those at risk for kidney disease should limit their use of NSAIDs and consult a healthcare provider for alternative pain management options.

2. High Sodium Intake:

Excessive sodium in the diet can raise blood pressure and increase the strain on the kidneys. Over time, high sodium intake can lead to the development of kidney disease or worsen existing kidney conditions. It is important to limit sodium consumption by avoiding processed foods, salty snacks, and fast food and instead opting for whole, unprocessed foods.

3.   Processed Foods High in Phosphorus:

Phosphorus is an essential mineral, but too much of it—especially in the form of inorganic phosphorus found in processed foods—can harm the kidneys. High phosphorus levels can lead to calcification in the kidneys, increasing the risk of kidney stones and worsening kidney function in individuals with CKD. It is best to limit foods such as soda, processed cheese, and deli meats, which are often high in inorganic phosphorus.

4.   Heavy Metals (Lead, Mercury, Cadmium):

Exposure to heavy metals, such as lead, mercury, and cadmium, can be highly toxic to the kidneys. These metals can accumulate in the body over time, leading to kidney damage and impaired detoxification. To minimise exposure, it is important to avoid contaminated water sources, limit the consumption of fish high in mercury, and reduce contact with heavy metal-laden industrial products.

5.   Excessive Alcohol Consumption:

Chronic heavy drinking can cause long-term damage to the kidneys. Alcohol acts as a diuretic, causing dehydration and forcing the kidneys to work harder to filter the blood. Over time, excessive alcohol consumption can lead to high blood pressure, a major risk factor for kidney disease. Limiting alcohol intake to moderate levels is essential for protecting kidney health.

By being mindful of these nephrotoxic substances and making lifestyle choices that support rather than harm the kidneys, individuals can significantly reduce their risk of developing kidney-related issues.

Case Study: Herbal Supplements Helped a 55-Year-Old Recover from Kidney Stress

Background: Linda, a 55-year-old woman, had been experiencing mild kidney stress for several years. Her doctor noted that her blood pressure was higher than normal, and routine blood tests revealed slightly elevated creatinine levels, indicating that her kidneys were under strain. Linda also reported occasional swelling in her ankles and hands, symptoms associated with fluid retention. Concerned about her long-term kidney health, Linda sought out a natural approach to support her kidneys and reduce the strain on her renal system.

Intervention: After consulting with a naturopathic practitioner, Linda was advised to incorporate several herbal supplements into her daily routine to support her kidneys and enhance detoxification. The practitioner recommended **dandelion** for its diuretic properties, which would help reduce her fluid retention and promote kidney detoxification. Linda was also prescribed **nettle** to reduce inflammation in her kidneys and support urine flow.

In addition to these herbs, Linda began taking **N-acetyl cysteine (NAC)** to protect her kidneys from oxidative stress and improve their ability to detoxify waste products. Her practitioner also advised her to reduce her sodium intake and avoid NSAIDs, which she had been taking frequently for joint pain.

Outcome: After three months of following her herbal supplement regimen, Linda noticed significant improvements in her kidney health. Her blood pressure began to normalise, and the swelling in her ankles and hands reduced. She also reported feeling more energised, with less fatigue and clearer thinking. Follow-up blood tests showed that her creatinine levels had returned to a healthy range, indicating that her kidneys were no longer under strain.

Linda's experience illustrates how herbal supplements like dandelion, nettle, and NAC can provide gentle, natural support for kidney health, especially in cases of mild kidney stress. By addressing the root causes of her kidney issues—such as fluid retention and inflammation—Linda was able to restore balance to her renal system and avoid further kidney damage.

Conclusion

Herbal supplements and phytochemicals offer a powerful and natural way to support kidney health and enhance the body's detoxification processes. With herbs like dandelion and nettle promoting kidney function and reducing inflammation, and nutraceuticals like NAC providing antioxidant protection, these remedies are valuable tools for maintaining kidney health. However, it is just as important to avoid nephrotoxic substances that can harm the kidneys and lead to long-term damage. By incorporating kidney-supportive herbs and making mindful lifestyle choices, individuals can protect their kidneys and ensure they function optimally for years to come.

Summary: Herbal Supplements and Phytochemicals for Kidney Detox

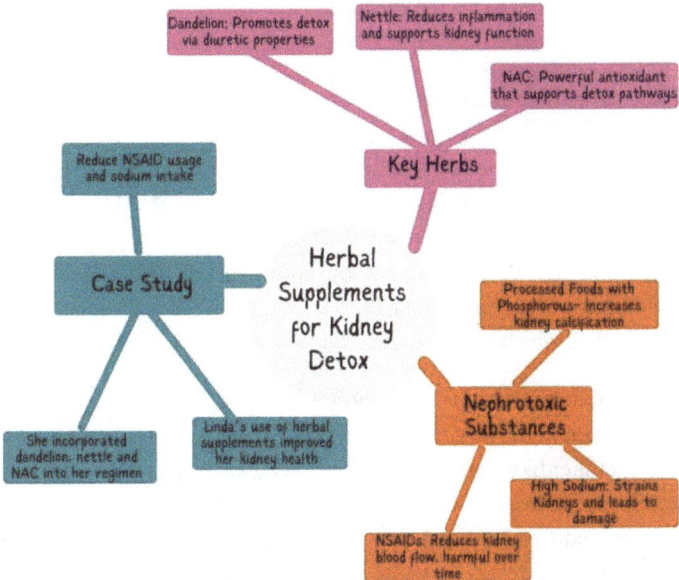

Dandelion: Promotes detox via diuretic properties

Nettle: Reduces inflammation and supports kidney function

NAC: Powerful antioxidant that supports detox pathways

Key Herbs

Reduce NSAID usage and sodium intake

Case Study

Herbal Supplements for Kidney Detox

Processed Foods with Phosphorous: Increases kidney calcification

Nephrotoxic Substances

She incorporated dandelion, nettle and NAC into her regimen

Linda's use of herbal supplements improved her kidney health

High Sodium: Strains kidneys and leads to damage

NSAIDs: Reduces kidney blood flow, harmful over time

Chapter 11
Exercise, Movement, and Kidney Function

How Physical Activity Supports Detoxification and Kidney Health

Physical activity is an essential component of maintaining overall health, and it plays a significant role in supporting the detoxification processes in the body, including kidney function. The kidneys are responsible for filtering toxins and waste from the bloodstream, maintaining fluid balance, and regulating electrolytes. Regular exercise helps enhance these functions by improving circulation, reducing inflammation, and promoting the movement of fluids throughout the body, all of which aid the kidneys in their role of detoxification.

When you engage in physical activity, your heart pumps more blood throughout the body, including to the kidneys, which allows them to filter blood more efficiently. Exercise also promotes sweating, another key mechanism for eliminating toxins through the skin, which in turn reduces the load on the kidneys. Additionally, by helping maintain a healthy body weight, exercise reduces the risk of conditions like high blood pressure and diabetes, which are major contributors to kidney disease.

Moreover, exercise stimulates the lymphatic system, which works alongside the kidneys to remove waste from the body. The lymphatic system relies on movement to function, as it doesn't have a pump like the cardiovascular system. Regular physical activity helps "pump" lymph fluid through the lymphatic vessels, allowing the body to dispose of toxins more effectively. This makes movement a crucial part of any detoxification routine and kidney health maintenance.

Types of Physical Activity That Benefit Kidney Health:

1. Aerobic Exercise:

Aerobic activities, such as walking, swimming, and cycling, increase your heart rate and improve cardiovascular health, which directly benefits the kidneys by enhancing blood flow. These exercises also help lower blood pressure and reduce the risk of kidney-related diseases.

2. Strength Training:

Building muscle through resistance exercises helps maintain a healthy metabolism and body composition. Strength training also improves insulin sensitivity, reducing the risk of diabetes, a major cause of kidney damage. Lifting weights or using resistance bands can be beneficial for overall kidney health, especially when performed in moderation.

3. Yoga and Stretching:

Yoga and stretching exercises support kidney health by promoting relaxation, reducing stress, and improving circulation to the kidneys. Certain yoga postures, such as **Paschimottanasana** (Seated Forward Bend) and **Ardha Matsyendrasana** (Half Lord of the Fishes Pose), target the abdominal and lower back areas, helping stimulate kidney function. Breathing techniques, such as **pranayama**, further enhance detoxification by oxygenating the blood and promoting relaxation.

4. Low-Impact Exercises:

For individuals with kidney disease or those who cannot engage in high-intensity workouts, low-impact exercises like tai chi, gentle yoga, and walking are excellent alternatives. These activities support kidney health by promoting circulation and reducing stress without placing additional strain on the body.

The Importance of Movement in Preventing Kidney Dysfunction

Staying physically active is key to preventing kidney dysfunction. A sedentary lifestyle is associated with numerous health risks, including obesity, high blood pressure, and type 2 diabetes, all of which are leading causes of chronic kidney disease (CKD). Lack of movement can also contribute to poor circulation and fluid retention, increasing the risk of kidney problems.

1. Reducing Blood Pressure and Improving Circulation:

Hypertension, or high blood pressure, is a major risk factor for kidney disease. Regular physical activity helps lower blood pressure by improving the elasticity of blood vessels, making it easier for the heart to pump blood through the body. When blood pressure is controlled, the kidneys are less likely to be damaged by excessive pressure on the delicate blood vessels within the kidneys.

2. Managing Blood Sugar Levels:

Physical activity helps regulate blood sugar levels by improving the body's sensitivity to insulin. When insulin sensitivity is improved, the body is better able to use glucose for energy, preventing spikes in blood sugar. This is crucial for kidney health, as elevated blood sugar levels can damage the kidneys over time, leading to diabetic nephropathy—a common complication of uncontrolled diabetes.

3. Promoting Weight Loss and Reducing Obesity:

Obesity increases the risk of kidney disease by placing extra strain on the kidneys, forcing them to work harder to filter waste and regulate fluids. Exercise helps prevent weight gain and promotes fat loss, reducing the workload on the kidneys and lowering the risk of kidney dysfunction.

4.   Preventing Inflammation and Oxidative Stress:

Chronic inflammation and oxidative stress are common in individuals with kidney disease and can lead to further kidney damage. Exercise has been shown to reduce inflammation by decreasing the production of pro-inflammatory cytokines and increasing antioxidant defences. By engaging in regular physical activity, individuals can reduce inflammation, protect their kidneys from further damage, and enhance their body's ability to detoxify.

5.   Improving Fluid Balance and Preventing Water Retention:

Regular movement helps promote the flow of fluids through the body, preventing fluid retention and swelling, which can be signs of kidney dysfunction. Exercise encourages the kidneys to regulate water balance more efficiently, ensuring that excess fluids are eliminated through urine rather than being retained in the body.

For individuals at risk of kidney disease or those looking to maintain healthy kidney function, incorporating movement into daily routines is essential. A combination of aerobic exercise, strength training, and mindful movement practices like yoga can help keep the kidneys functioning optimally and reduce the risk of kidney-related issues.

Case Study: A 70-Year-Old Maintains Kidney Health with Regular Walking and Yoga

Background: Margaret, a 70-year-old retiree, had been dealing with high blood pressure for several years. She was concerned about her kidney health, as her doctor had mentioned that her creatinine levels were higher than normal, indicating that her kidneys might be under strain. Margaret also experienced occasional swelling in her legs and ankles, a sign of fluid retention. After discussing her concerns with her doctor, she decided to incorporate more physical activity into her daily routine to improve her overall health and protect her kidneys.

Intervention: Margaret began by introducing regular walking into her routine, starting with 20-minute walks around her neighbourhood three times a week. Walking is a low-impact aerobic exercise that helps improve circulation, reduce blood pressure, and promote fluid movement, making it ideal for supporting kidney health.

In addition to walking, Margaret also joined a local yoga class for seniors, where she learned gentle yoga postures and breathing exercises. Her yoga instructor taught her poses that specifically targeted the kidneys and promoted relaxation, such as **Setu Bandhasana** (Bridge Pose) and **Supta Baddha Konasana** (Reclining Bound Angle Pose). These postures helped reduce the swelling in her legs and encouraged better kidney function. The breathing exercises, or **pranayama**, helped Margaret reduce stress, which had been contributing to her high blood pressure.

Outcome: After three months of regular walking and yoga, Margaret noticed significant improvements in her overall health. Her blood pressure decreased, and her doctor noted that her creatinine levels had stabilised, indicating that her kidneys were no longer under as much strain. The swelling in her legs had reduced, and she felt more energised and less fatigued. Margaret also enjoyed the mental clarity and relaxation that yoga provided, helping her manage stress more effectively.

Margaret's experience highlights how even gentle forms of exercise, such as walking and yoga, can have a profound impact on kidney health, especially for older adults. By staying active, reducing stress, and promoting fluid balance, Margaret was able to support her kidneys and prevent further decline in function.

Conclusion

Exercise and movement play a crucial role in supporting kidney function and detoxification. Whether through aerobic activities, strength training, or mindful movement practices like yoga, regular physical activity helps improve circulation, reduce inflammation, and promote the elimination of toxins from the body. For individuals at risk of kidney disease or those looking to maintain healthy kidney function, incorporating movement into daily life is an essential step in protecting the kidneys and promoting overall well-being.

Margaret's case demonstrates the power of simple lifestyle changes—such as regular walking and yoga—in maintaining kidney health, even in older adults. By staying active and mindful of fluid balance, you can support your kidneys in their vital role of filtering waste and keeping the body in balance.

Summary: Exercise, Movement, and Kidney Function

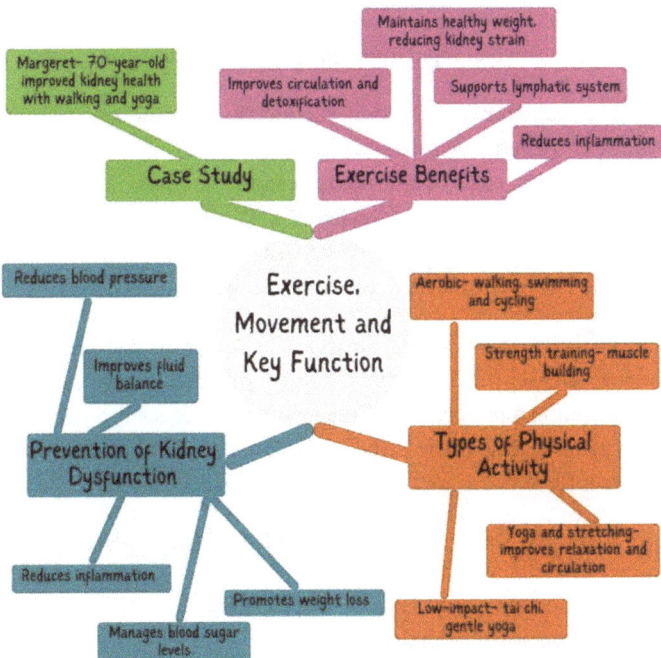

Chapter 12
Intravenous (IV) Drip
Therapy for Kidney Health

Understanding IV Drip Therapy and Its Uses

Intravenous (IV) drip therapy is a method of delivering fluids, vitamins, minerals, and other nutrients directly into the bloodstream, bypassing the digestive system. This allows for faster absorption and immediate access to essential nutrients that can support various functions of the body, including kidney health. IV therapy is often used in clinical settings for rehydration, detoxification, and replenishment of nutrients, especially when oral supplementation is insufficient or when rapid intervention is required.

For individuals with kidney concerns, IV therapy can offer significant benefits by providing hydration, reducing oxidative stress, and supporting the body's detoxification pathways. By delivering nutrients directly into the bloodstream, IV therapy ensures that the kidneys have the resources they need to filter blood effectively, maintain electrolyte balance, and eliminate waste products.

IV drip therapy can also be useful for people dealing with chronic kidney disease (CKD), where kidney function is impaired, and detoxification is less efficient. Certain IV therapies, such as glutathione and vitamin C drips, help protect the kidneys from oxidative damage, reduce inflammation, and improve overall kidney function.

When IV Drip Therapy is Used for Kidney Health:

- To rapidly rehydrate the body in cases of dehydration, which can strain the kidneys.
- To replenish depleted levels of essential vitamins and minerals, such as B vitamins, magnesium, and vitamin C, which support kidney function.
- To reduce oxidative stress and inflammation in the kidneys, helping protect against long-term damage.

- To improve circulation and detoxification, reducing the buildup of waste products that the kidneys must filter.

Types of IV Drips that Benefit the Kidneys

There are several types of IV drips that specifically support kidney health, each offering unique benefits based on the nutrients they deliver. Among the most beneficial IV therapies for kidney health are **glutathione**, **vitamin C**, and **hydration drips**.

1.   Glutathione Drip

Glutathione is one of the body's most powerful antioxidants, playing a crucial role in neutralising free radicals and protecting cells from oxidative stress. For the kidneys, which are constantly filtering blood and removing toxins, glutathione is essential in minimising damage caused by harmful substances. IV glutathione therapy delivers this antioxidant directly into the bloodstream, bypassing the digestive system and allowing for rapid absorption and utilisation by the kidneys.

a.   How it benefits the kidneys:

Glutathione helps protect kidney cells from damage caused by toxins, medications, and other harmful substances. It supports the detoxification process by enhancing the body's ability to eliminate toxins, which reduces the workload on the kidneys. For individuals with chronic kidney disease or those at risk of kidney damage, glutathione can help slow the progression of kidney dysfunction by reducing oxidative stress.

b.   Common use:

Glutathione IV drips are often administered as part of a comprehensive detoxification or antioxidant therapy protocol. They may be recommended for individuals with early-stage CKD, those exposed to nephrotoxic medications, or anyone looking to enhance their body's natural detox pathways.

2.   Vitamin C Drip

Vitamin C is a potent antioxidant and immune booster that supports various functions in the body, including kidney health. As a water-soluble vitamin, vitamin C is easily filtered by the kidneys and plays a key role in protecting kidney tissues from oxidative damage. High-dose IV vitamin C is especially beneficial for reducing inflammation and supporting the immune system, both of which are important for maintaining healthy kidney function.

a.   How it benefits the kidneys:

Vitamin C helps reduce inflammation in the kidneys, which can occur due to infections, high blood pressure, or exposure to toxins. It also supports collagen production, which is important for maintaining the integrity of kidney tissues. By reducing oxidative stress, vitamin C protects the kidneys from damage that can lead to kidney disease or further decline in kidney function.

b.   Common use:

IV vitamin C is often used in detoxification protocols or as part of supportive therapy for individuals with chronic health conditions. It is particularly useful for individuals with kidney issues, as it enhances antioxidant defences and supports overall kidney health.

3.   Hydration Drip (Saline or Lactated Ringer's Solution)

Proper hydration is essential for kidney health, as the kidneys rely on an adequate supply of water to filter blood, eliminate waste, and maintain electrolyte balance. **Hydration drips** typically contain saline or lactated Ringer's solution, both of which help replenish fluids and electrolytes in the body. IV hydration is particularly beneficial for individuals who are dehydrated, as it provides immediate rehydration without relying on the digestive system.

a.   How it benefits the kidneys:

Hydration drips help restore fluid balance, which reduces the risk of kidney stones, improves urine flow, and supports the kidneys in flushing out toxins more effectively. For individuals with CKD or those at risk of kidney disease, maintaining proper hydration is key to preventing further kidney damage and ensuring that the kidneys function optimally.

b.   Common use:

Hydration drips are commonly used in hospitals and clinics to treat dehydration, especially in individuals who are unable to drink sufficient fluids. They are also used as part of detoxification protocols to support the kidneys in eliminating waste and toxins more efficiently.

Case Study: A 50-Year-Old Man Uses IV Therapy to Stabilise Early-Stage CKD

Background: James, a 50-year-old man, was diagnosed with early-stage chronic kidney disease (CKD) during a routine medical checkup. His doctor noted that his creatinine levels were elevated, and his glomerular filtration rate (GFR) had started to decline, indicating that his kidneys were under strain. James had a history of high blood pressure, which likely contributed to his kidney issues. Concerned about his long-term kidney health, James sought out additional therapies to help stabilise his kidney function and slow the progression of CKD.

Intervention: After consulting with a naturopathic doctor, James was introduced to IV therapy as a supportive treatment for his kidneys. He began receiving a combination of **glutathione** and **vitamin C** IV drips twice a month to reduce oxidative stress and support his kidneys' detoxification processes. His doctor also recommended **hydration drips** to ensure that he remained properly hydrated, as dehydration could exacerbate his kidney issues.

The glutathione IV drips were designed to protect James' kidney cells from oxidative damage, while the vitamin C drips provided additional antioxidant support and reduced inflammation. The hydration drips helped maintain his fluid balance and encouraged his kidneys to flush out toxins more efficiently.

Outcome: After three months of regular IV therapy, James' kidney function stabilised. His creatinine levels decreased slightly, and his GFR improved, indicating that his kidneys were functioning more efficiently. James also reported feeling more energised and less fatigued, and he noticed that his blood pressure was more stable as well. His doctor was pleased with the results and recommended continuing the IV therapy as part of a long-term strategy to support his kidney health.

James' case highlights the potential benefits of IV drip therapy for individuals with early-stage CKD or those at risk of kidney disease. By providing the kidneys with essential antioxidants and ensuring proper hydration, IV therapy can help stabilise kidney function and protect against further damage.

Conclusion

Intravenous (IV) drip therapy offers a valuable tool for supporting kidney health, especially for individuals dealing with kidney stress or early-stage CKD. Glutathione and vitamin C drips help reduce oxidative stress and protect kidney tissues from damage, while hydration drips ensure that the kidneys have the fluids they need to function optimally. By delivering essential nutrients directly into the bloodstream, IV therapy bypasses the digestive system and provides immediate benefits, making it a highly effective option for enhancing kidney health and detoxification.

James' case demonstrates how IV drip therapy can help stabilise kidney function and improve overall health, particularly for individuals with compromised kidney function. For those looking to protect their kidneys and support their body's detoxification processes, IV therapy can be a powerful addition to a comprehensive kidney health plan.

Summary: Intravenous (IV) Drip Therapy for Kidney Health

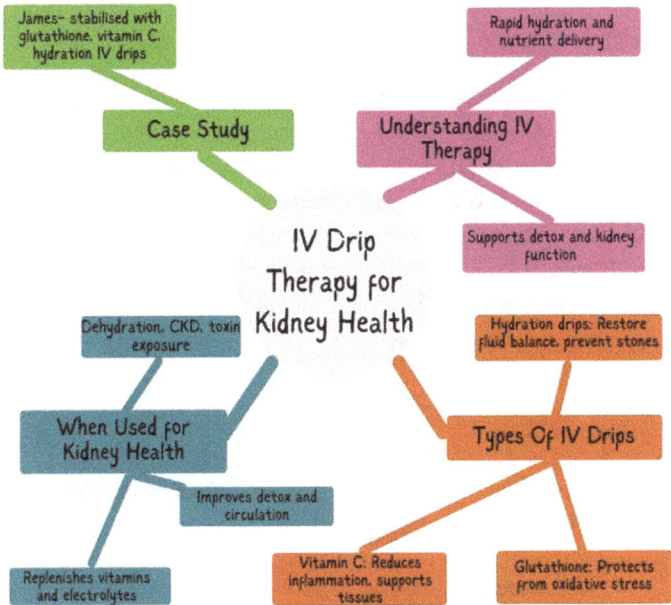

IV Drip Therapy for Kidney Health

- Case Study
  - James– stabilised with glutathione, vitamin C, hydration IV drips

- Understanding IV Therapy
  - Rapid hydration and nutrient delivery
  - Supports detox and kidney function

- When Used for Kidney Health
  - Dehydration, CKD, toxin exposure
  - Improves detox and circulation
  - Replenishes vitamins and electrolytes

- Types Of IV Drips
  - Hydration drips: Restore fluid balance, prevent stones
  - Vitamin C: Reduces inflammation, supports tissues
  - Glutathione: Protects from oxidative stress

Chapter 13
Chronic Kidney Disease (CKD) and Detoxification Challenges

Understanding CKD and Its Effects on Kidney Function

Chronic Kidney Disease (CKD) is a long-term condition in which the kidneys gradually lose their ability to filter waste, regulate fluid balance, and maintain essential electrolytes. This progressive loss of kidney function can lead to a dangerous buildup of waste products in the body, causing complications such as high blood pressure, anaemia, weak bones, poor nutritional health, and nerve damage. CKD is classified into five stages, ranging from mild kidney impairment (stage 1) to complete kidney failure (stage 5, also known as end-stage renal disease or ESRD).

Causes of CKD:

CKD is most commonly caused by conditions that put long-term stress on the kidneys, such as:

- **Diabetes:** High blood sugar levels damage the blood vessels in the kidneys, reducing their ability to filter waste and regulate fluids.

- **Hypertension (High Blood Pressure):** Elevated blood pressure damages the small blood vessels in the kidneys over time, leading to reduced kidney function.

- **Glomerulonephritis:** Inflammation of the kidney's filtering units, which can lead to scarring and permanent damage.

- **Polycystic Kidney Disease (PKD):** A genetic condition where fluid-filled cysts grow in the kidneys, eventually leading to kidney failure.

As kidney function declines in CKD, patients face increasing challenges with detoxification. The kidneys are responsible for filtering waste products like urea and creatinine from the bloodstream, regulating electrolytes (e.g., sodium, potassium), and maintaining the body's acid-base balance. When these functions are impaired, toxic substances accumulate in the body, leading to a wide range of health issues, including fatigue, swelling, shortness of breath, and cognitive impairment.

Symptoms of CKD Include:

- Fatigue and weakness
- Swelling in the legs, ankles, or feet (oedema)
- Shortness of breath
- Confusion or difficulty concentrating
- Nausea and loss of appetite
- Frequent urination, particularly at night
- High blood pressure that is difficult to control

By the time CKD progresses to its later stages, the kidneys are significantly impaired, and patients may require dialysis or a kidney transplant to survive. However, in the earlier stages, there are many strategies to slow the progression of CKD and support kidney health, including dietary changes, exercise, and supportive therapies.

How to Support Kidney Health in CKD with Diet, Exercise, and Therapies

For individuals diagnosed with CKD, there are several lifestyle interventions and therapies that can help manage symptoms, improve kidney function, and slow the progression of the disease. These approaches focus on reducing the kidneys' workload, supporting overall detoxification, and addressing the underlying causes of CKD, such as hypertension and diabetes.

1. Dietary Support for CKD

Diet plays a crucial role in managing CKD and supporting kidney health. A kidney-friendly diet focuses on reducing the intake of substances that the kidneys must filter, such as protein, sodium, potassium, and phosphorus, while ensuring that the body receives essential nutrients to maintain overall health.

- Reduce Protein Intake:

High-protein diets place additional strain on the kidneys, as they must work harder to eliminate waste products from protein metabolism. For individuals with CKD, reducing protein intake can help lessen the kidneys' workload. Instead of focusing on animal-based proteins (meat, dairy, eggs), patients can incorporate plant-based proteins, such as lentils, quinoa, and tofu, which are easier on the kidneys.

- Limit Sodium and Potassium:

Sodium and potassium are two key electrolytes that the kidneys regulate. In CKD, it becomes more difficult for the kidneys to manage these electrolytes, leading to imbalances that can cause swelling, high blood pressure, and heart problems. Patients are often advised to limit their sodium intake to under 2,300 mg per day and avoid high-potassium foods like bananas, potatoes, and tomatoes.

- Control Phosphorus Levels:

Elevated phosphorus levels can cause calcium to leach from the bones, leading to weakened bones and an increased risk of fractures. Foods high in phosphorus, such as dairy products, processed meats, and soda, should be limited. Some individuals may also require phosphorus binders to help control phosphorus levels in the blood.

- Increase Hydration:

Maintaining adequate hydration is essential for kidney health, but fluid intake should be balanced based on individual needs. Drinking too little water can lead to dehydration and strain the kidneys, while drinking too much can lead to fluid retention, especially in advanced CKD. Patients should work with their healthcare providers to determine the right level of hydration for their condition.

2.   Exercise and Movement for CKD

Regular physical activity is beneficial for individuals with CKD, as it helps improve circulation, lower blood pressure, and manage blood sugar levels, all of which are critical for protecting kidney function. Exercise also promotes detoxification by enhancing lymphatic flow and reducing inflammation throughout the body.

• Aerobic Exercise:

Activities like walking, swimming, and cycling improve cardiovascular health, which supports the kidneys by increasing blood flow and reducing the risk of hypertension and diabetes. Even moderate exercise can have a significant impact on kidney function by improving overall health and reducing risk factors for CKD.

• Strength Training:

Resistance exercises help maintain muscle mass and metabolism, which are often compromised in individuals with CKD. Strength training can also improve insulin sensitivity, reducing the risk of diabetic kidney damage.

• Gentle Movement (Yoga, Tai Chi):

Yoga and tai chi are excellent forms of exercise for individuals with CKD, as they help reduce stress, improve flexibility, and promote relaxation. Certain yoga postures, such as twists and forward bends, can stimulate kidney function and support detoxification.

3.   Supportive Therapies for CKD

In addition to lifestyle changes, various therapies can help support kidney health and reduce the progression of CKD. These therapies include:

- IV Drip Therapy:

For individuals with CKD, IV hydration therapy can help maintain proper fluid balance and prevent dehydration, which can exacerbate kidney problems. IV drips containing antioxidants like glutathione or vitamin C can also protect the kidneys from oxidative stress and inflammation.

- Acupuncture:

Acupuncture is a traditional Chinese medicine practice that has been used to treat kidney-related issues for centuries. By stimulating specific points on the body, acupuncture helps improve circulation, reduce stress, and promote the kidneys' detoxification processes.

- Herbal Supplements:

Herbal remedies like dandelion and nettle can be used to support kidney function by promoting urine production and reducing inflammation. However, it is essential to consult with a healthcare provider before using herbal supplements, as some herbs may interact with medications or be harmful in advanced CKD.

Case Study: How a 65-Year-Old Man Managed CKD Through Lifestyle Changes

Background: Paul, a 65-year-old man, had been managing type 2 diabetes and high blood pressure for over a decade. During a routine checkup, his doctor noted that his creatinine levels were elevated, and his glomerular filtration rate (GFR) had dropped to 45, indicating stage 3 CKD. Paul was concerned about his kidney health, as both his father and grandfather had experienced kidney failure in their later years. Wanting to avoid dialysis, Paul sought ways to improve his kidney function naturally through lifestyle changes.

Intervention: Paul's doctor referred him to a nephrologist, who advised him to make dietary changes to support his kidneys. He was instructed to reduce his protein intake and switch to more plant-based sources of protein, such as beans, lentils, and quinoa. He also cut back on sodium and processed foods, opting instead for fresh vegetables, whole grains, and low-sodium alternatives. Paul's doctor also recommended limiting high-potassium foods like bananas and tomatoes to prevent electrolyte imbalances.

In addition to dietary changes, Paul began exercising regularly. He took up walking for 30 minutes a day and practised gentle yoga to reduce stress and improve circulation. The yoga poses, such as **Paschimottanasana** (Seated Forward Bend) and **Setu Bandhasana** (Bridge Pose), helped him relax and focus on deep breathing, which supported his overall well-being.

To further support his kidneys, Paul started IV drip therapy, receiving hydration drips to ensure that he remained properly hydrated and glutathione drips to protect his kidneys from oxidative stress. He also took a daily supplement of NAC (N-acetyl cysteine) to support his body's detoxification processes.

Outcome: After six months of making these lifestyle changes, Paul saw a marked improvement in his kidney health. His GFR increased to 55, and his creatinine levels decreased, indicating that his kidneys were functioning more efficiently. He also experienced more energy, reduced swelling in his legs, and better control of his blood pressure. His nephrologist was pleased with the progress and advised him to continue his new regimen to maintain kidney health.

Paul's case illustrates how lifestyle changes—combined with supportive therapies—can have a profound impact on managing CKD and preventing further kidney damage. By adopting a kidney-friendly diet, exercising regularly, and incorporating IV therapy and supplements, Paul was able to stabilise his CKD and improve his quality of life.

Conclusion

Chronic Kidney Disease (CKD) presents significant challenges in terms of detoxification and overall health, but with the right interventions, it is possible to slow the progression of the disease and support kidney function. A combination of diet, exercise, and therapies such as IV drip therapy, acupuncture, and herbal supplements can help reduce the strain on the kidneys and improve detoxification pathways. Paul's case demonstrates how adopting these changes can have a lasting positive impact on kidney health, even in the later stages of CKD.

Summary: Chronic Kidney Disease (CKD) and Detoxification Challenges

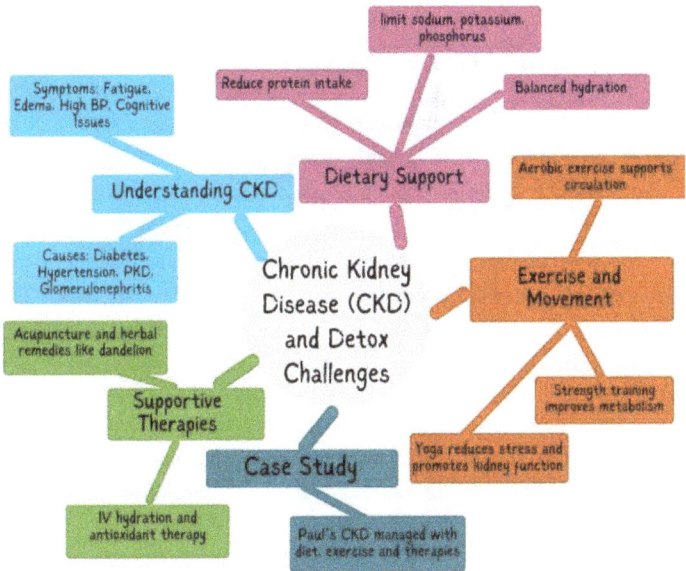

Chapter 14
Modern Medical Perspectives on Kidney Detox

The Role of Conventional Medicine in Kidney Health

Conventional medicine plays an essential role in diagnosing, managing, and treating kidney-related health issues, particularly when it comes to conditions like Chronic Kidney Disease (CKD), acute kidney injury (AKI), and other disorders that impair kidney function. While holistic approaches like diet, exercise, and supplements can offer significant benefits, conventional medicine provides the diagnostic tools and therapeutic interventions needed to monitor kidney health and manage more severe cases of kidney dysfunction.

The kidneys are vital organs responsible for filtering waste products from the blood, balancing electrolytes, regulating blood pressure, and maintaining the body's fluid balance. When the kidneys fail to perform these functions efficiently, waste products like urea, creatinine, and excess electrolytes accumulate in the bloodstream, leading to a range of health problems.

Conventional medicine typically approaches kidney health through a combination of diagnostic tests, medications, and, in more severe cases, dialysis or kidney transplantation. These interventions are necessary when kidney function declines beyond a certain point, as untreated kidney failure can be life-threatening.

Diagnostic Tools for Monitoring Kidney Health:

1.   Blood Tests (Creatinine and Glomerular Filtration Rate - GFR):

Blood tests are the primary way that healthcare providers assess kidney function. **Creatinine** is a waste product produced by muscles, and its levels in the blood indicate how well the kidneys are filtering it out. **GFR** is a calculation based on creatinine levels that estimates how efficiently the kidneys are functioning. A lower GFR indicates reduced kidney function and is used to stage Chronic Kidney Disease (CKD).

2.   Urine Tests (Protein and Albumin):

Urine tests can detect the presence of **protein** or **albumin** in the urine, both of which are signs of kidney damage. When the kidneys are functioning properly, they filter out waste but retain proteins. The presence of protein in the urine (proteinuria) is an early marker of kidney disease.

3.   Imaging Tests (Ultrasound, CT Scan, MRI):

Imaging tests allow doctors to visualise the kidneys and assess their size, shape, and structure. Ultrasound is often used to detect blockages, cysts, or tumors that may be affecting kidney function. In some cases, a **CT scan** or **MRI** may be used to provide a more detailed view of the kidneys.

4.   Kidney Biopsy:

A kidney biopsy involves taking a small sample of kidney tissue for examination under a microscope. This test is typically used to diagnose specific kidney conditions, such as glomerulonephritis or nephrotic syndrome, and to assess the severity of kidney damage.

How Medical Tests Can Help Monitor Kidney Function

Regular monitoring of kidney function is essential for detecting kidney disease in its early stages and preventing further damage. Medical tests, such as those mentioned above, allow healthcare providers to track changes in kidney function over time and adjust treatment plans accordingly.

1.   Detecting Early-Stage Kidney Disease:

Many kidney conditions, such as CKD, do not present symptoms until significant damage has occurred. Regular blood and urine tests can help identify kidney disease in its early stages, even before symptoms develop. Early detection is critical, as it allows for lifestyle modifications and treatments that can slow or even halt the progression of kidney disease.

2.   Monitoring Disease Progression:

For individuals already diagnosed with CKD or other kidney conditions, routine testing is essential for monitoring the disease's progression. By tracking GFR, creatinine, and protein levels, healthcare providers can determine how well the kidneys are functioning and adjust medications or therapies to protect kidney function.

3.   Guiding Treatment Decisions:

Medical tests help guide treatment decisions by providing objective data on kidney function. For example, elevated creatinine levels may prompt a healthcare provider to adjust medications, while worsening proteinuria may indicate the need for more aggressive treatment. In some cases, medical tests can also determine whether a patient needs dialysis or a kidney transplant.

Balancing Modern and Holistic Approaches to Kidney Health

While conventional medicine provides vital tools for diagnosing and treating kidney disease, a holistic approach that includes diet, lifestyle changes, and natural therapies can complement medical treatments and enhance kidney health. By combining modern medical interventions with holistic practices, individuals can take a proactive approach to their kidney health and reduce the risk of complications.

Medications Commonly Used in Kidney Disease:

1.   ACE Inhibitors and ARBs:

These medications are used to lower blood pressure and protect kidney function, especially in individuals with diabetes or hypertension. **Angiotensin-converting enzyme (ACE) inhibitors** and

angiotensin II receptor blockers (ARBs) help reduce proteinuria and slow the progression of CKD.

2.   Diuretics:

Diuretics help reduce fluid retention by increasing urine output, which can relieve swelling (oedema) and lower blood pressure. While helpful in manageing symptoms, diuretics must be carefully monitored to avoid dehydration, which can worsen kidney function.

3.   Phosphate Binders:

In advanced CKD, the kidneys may struggle to regulate phosphate levels, leading to an excess of phosphate in the blood. Phosphate binders are medications that prevent the absorption of phosphorus from food, helping to maintain normal phosphate levels and protect the bones and cardiovascular system.

4.   Erythropoietin (EPO) and Iron Supplements:

Individuals with CKD often develop anaemia due to reduced production of **erythropoietin (EPO)**, a hormone that stimulates red blood cell production. EPO injections and iron supplements can help treat anaemia and improve energy levels in individuals with kidney disease.

Complementary Therapies to Support Kidney Health:

In addition to medications, complementary therapies can play a key role in supporting kidney function and improving overall health. Some of the most effective complementary therapies include:

1.   Dietary Changes:

A kidney-friendly diet can help reduce the strain on the kidneys and improve overall health. Reducing sodium, potassium, and phosphorus intake, while incorporating antioxidant-rich foods, can slow the progression of kidney disease.

2. Hydration Therapy:

Proper hydration supports the kidneys in filtering waste and maintaining fluid balance. However, individuals with advanced kidney disease should consult their healthcare provider to determine appropriate fluid intake, as too much fluid can lead to swelling and heart issues.

3. Herbal Supplements and Antioxidants:

Herbal supplements such as dandelion, nettle, and turmeric have been shown to support kidney function by reducing inflammation and promoting detoxification. Antioxidants, such as **N-acetyl cysteine (NAC)** and glutathione, help protect the kidneys from oxidative stress and free radical damage.

4. Stress Management (Yoga, Meditation, Acupuncture):

Chronic stress can contribute to high blood pressure and kidney damage. Stress management techniques like yoga, meditation, and acupuncture can help reduce stress and improve circulation, which benefits kidney function. Yoga, in particular, has been shown to lower blood pressure and promote relaxation, both of which are essential for kidney health.

Conclusion

Modern medical perspectives on kidney detoxification emphasise the importance of regular monitoring, medications, and lifestyle interventions in maintaining kidney health. Diagnostic tests such as blood, urine, and imaging studies provide critical insights into kidney function, allowing healthcare providers to detect early signs of kidney disease, monitor its progression, and tailor treatment plans accordingly.

By combining conventional medical treatments with holistic practices like dietary changes, hydration therapy, and stress management, individuals can support their kidney health and reduce the risk of long-term complications. Whether through medications, IV drips, or lifestyle modifications, balancing modern and holistic approaches offers the best opportunity for maintaining optimal kidney function and overall well-being.

Summary: Modern Medical Perspectives on Kidney Detox

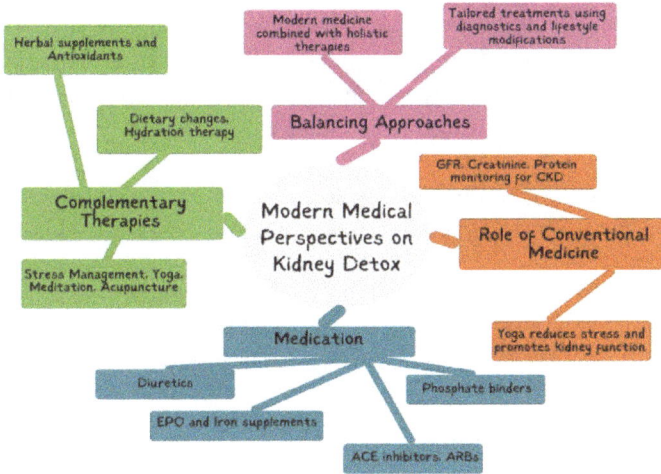

Chapter 15
Preventive Measures for Long-Term Kidney Health

Practical Steps for Protecting Your Kidneys Over Time

Maintaining healthy kidneys is crucial for overall well-being, as they are essential for filtering waste, regulating fluid balance, and maintaining electrolyte levels. Given the kidneys' vital role, it is important to adopt preventive strategies to safeguard their function over the long term. Many kidney issues, such as Chronic Kidney Disease (CKD) or Acute Kidney Injury (AKI), develop gradually over time, often due to lifestyle factors such as poor diet, dehydration, or the overuse of medications. By taking proactive steps now, you can reduce the risk of kidney dysfunction and promote long-term health.

Here are several key preventive measures that can help protect your kidneys and ensure they function optimally throughout your life:

1. Stay Hydrated

    Drinking adequate amounts of water is one of the simplest and most effective ways to support kidney health. Proper hydration helps the kidneys filter waste and toxins from the bloodstream while preventing the formation of kidney stones. While the general recommendation is to drink at least 8 glasses (2 litres) of water daily, individual needs vary based on age, activity level, and climate.

    a. **Tip:** Check the colour of your urine—pale yellow is a good indicator of adequate hydration. Darker urine suggests that you need to increase your fluid intake.

2. Eat a Balanced, Kidney-Friendly Diet

    Your diet plays a significant role in maintaining healthy kidneys. A balanced diet rich in fruits, vegetables, whole grains, and lean proteins supports overall kidney function and prevents kidney strain.

a. **Reduce Salt Intake:** Excessive sodium (salt) can lead to high blood pressure, which damages the small blood vessels in the kidneys. Aim to consume no more than 2,300 milligrams of sodium per day.

b. **Limit Processed Foods:** Processed foods often contain high levels of sodium, phosphorus, and unhealthy fats, all of which can be harmful to the kidneys. Opt for fresh, whole foods as much as possible.

c. **Maintain Proper Protein Intake:** While protein is essential for overall health, too much protein—especially from animal sources—can burden the kidneys. Moderate your intake and incorporate plant-based proteins like beans, lentils, and tofu.

d. **Include Kidney-Friendly Foods:** Foods such as berries, apples, cabbage, and cauliflower are low in potassium and phosphorus, making them ideal for kidney health.

3. Manage Blood Pressure and Blood Sugar Levels

High blood pressure and diabetes are two of the leading causes of kidney disease. Manageing these conditions is crucial for long-term kidney health.

a. **Monitor Blood Pressure:** Aim to keep your blood pressure below 120/80 mmHg. If you have hypertension, work with your healthcare provider to manage it through lifestyle changes and, if necessary, medications.

b. **Control Blood Sugar:** If you have diabetes or prediabetes, monitor your blood sugar levels regularly. Keep your blood sugar within your target range by following a healthy diet, exercising, and taking prescribed medications.

4. Exercise Regularly

Regular physical activity improves circulation, helps maintain a healthy weight, and reduces the risk of conditions that can harm the kidneys, such as hypertension and diabetes.

    a. **Tip:** Aim for at least 150 minutes of moderate-intensity aerobic exercise each week, such as brisk walking, swimming, or cycling. Incorporating strength training exercises at least twice a week can further support muscle health and metabolism.

5. Avoid Overuse of Medications

Certain over-the-counter medications, particularly **non-steroidal anti-inflammatory drugs (NSAIDs)** like ibuprofen and naproxen, can be harmful to the kidneys if used frequently or in high doses.

    a. **Tip:** If you experience chronic pain or inflammation, discuss safer alternatives with your healthcare provider to reduce the risk of kidney damage.

6. Quit Smoking

Smoking narrows blood vessels, reducing blood flow to the kidneys and impairing their ability to function properly. It also increases the risk of developing kidney disease. Quitting smoking improves circulation, reduces inflammation, and helps protect kidney health over time.

7. Limit Alcohol Consumption

Excessive alcohol intake can cause dehydration and strain the kidneys, leading to long-term damage.

    a. **Tip:** Limit alcohol consumption to moderate levels—no more than one drink per day for women and two drinks per day for men.

Early Detection and Preventive Screenings for Kidney Health

Regular check-ups and screenings are essential for detecting kidney problems early, before they become more serious. Early detection allows for timely interventions that can slow or prevent further damage. Even if you feel healthy, routine kidney function tests can reveal important information about your kidney health.

1.   Blood Tests (Creatinine and GFR)

A simple blood test can measure your **creatinine** levels and estimate your **glomerular filtration rate (GFR)**, which indicates how well your kidneys are filtering waste. A lower GFR suggests reduced kidney function, even if you are not experiencing symptoms. Regular blood tests can help track changes in kidney function over time.

2.   Urine Tests (Protein, Albumin)

Urine tests can detect **proteinuria**, or protein in the urine, which is an early sign of kidney damage. The presence of protein or **albumin** in the urine suggests that the kidneys' filtering units are damaged. Urine tests are particularly important for individuals with high blood pressure or diabetes, as they are at higher risk for kidney disease.

3.   Imaging Tests

Ultrasounds and other imaging tests can detect structural abnormalities in the kidneys, such as cysts, tumours, or blockages. Imaging tests are useful for diagnosing conditions like polycystic kidney disease (PKD) or kidney stones.

4.   Regular Monitoring for At-Risk Individuals

If you have risk factors for kidney disease, such as diabetes, hypertension, or a family history of kidney problems, regular monitoring is critical. Your healthcare provider may recommend more frequent screenings to catch any signs of kidney dysfunction early.

Case Study: A 40-Year-Old Woman Avoids Kidney Disease Through Preventive Measures

Background: Lena, a 40-year-old woman with a family history of kidney disease, was concerned about her long-term kidney health. Her father had developed CKD in his 50s, and she wanted to take proactive steps to avoid the same fate. Though Lena was generally healthy, she had high blood pressure and was overweight, both of which increased her risk of kidney disease.

Intervention: After discussing her concerns with her doctor, Lena decided to make lifestyle changes to protect her kidneys. She started by adopting a **low-sodium, kidney-friendly diet**, focusing on whole grains, fresh vegetables, and lean proteins. She significantly reduced her intake of processed foods and began cooking most of her meals at home. Lena also increased her water intake, aiming to drink 8–10 glasses of water per day.

Lena incorporated regular exercise into her routine, starting with brisk walking for 30 minutes a day and gradually adding strength training exercises twice a week. To manage her blood pressure, Lena worked with her doctor to adjust her medications and monitored her blood pressure at home. She also made an effort to reduce stress by practising mindfulness meditation and yoga.

Outcome: After six months of making these changes, Lena lost 15 pounds, her blood pressure stabilised within a healthy range, and her kidney function remained normal, as confirmed by blood and urine tests. Her doctor was pleased with her progress and encouraged her to continue with her preventive strategies.

Lena's proactive approach not only helped her avoid kidney disease but also improved her overall health and well-being. By making small but consistent lifestyle changes, she was able to reduce her risk of CKD and take control of her long-term kidney health.

Conclusion

Preventing kidney disease requires a combination of healthy lifestyle habits, regular screenings, and proactive measures to address risk factors like high blood pressure and diabetes. Staying hydrated, eating a balanced diet, exercising regularly, and avoiding harmful substances like NSAIDs, tobacco, and excessive alcohol are all essential for maintaining kidney function over the long term. Regular monitoring and early detection are key to catching any signs of kidney dysfunction before they become serious.

Lena's case shows how taking preventive steps can have a profound impact on kidney health and overall wellness. By following these practical guidelines, you can protect your kidneys and ensure they continue to function optimally for years to come.

Summary: Preventive Measures for Long-Term Kidney Health

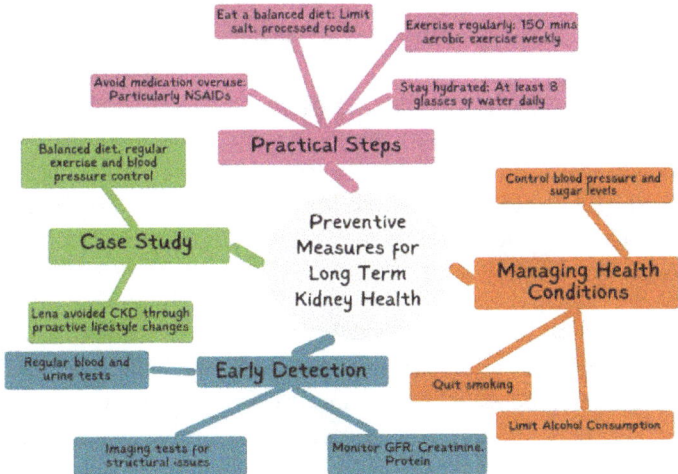

Chapter 16
Case Histories in Kidney Cleansing

Real-Life Stories of Individuals Who Improved Their Kidney Health Using Holistic Approaches

Holistic approaches to kidney health—encompassing diet, lifestyle changes, herbal supplements, and complementary therapies—can significantly impact kidney function and overall well-being. This chapter highlights real-life case histories of individuals who improved their kidney health using a combination of natural and conventional strategies. These stories illustrate how different age groups and health profiles can benefit from proactive kidney care, offering valuable insights into personalised approaches for detoxification and kidney support.

Case History 1: A 35-Year-Old Athlete with Recurrent Kidney Stones

Background: Sarah, a 35-year-old competitive marathon runner, had been dealing with recurrent kidney stones for several years. She experienced intense pain during stone passage and had undergone two procedures to remove larger stones. Despite following conventional medical advice, her kidney stones kept coming back. Sarah's doctors advised her to stay hydrated, but her physically demanding training schedule often left her dehydrated, which contributed to the formation of kidney stones.

Intervention: After her third kidney stone episode, Sarah decided to take a more holistic approach to prevent future stones. She consulted a naturopathic doctor who recommended increasing her water intake to 3 litres per day to keep her kidneys well-hydrated, particularly during long training sessions. Additionally, Sarah adopted a **low-oxalate diet**, reducing her intake of foods like spinach, beets, and nuts, which are known to contribute to stone formation.

Her naturopath also recommended taking a **magnesium citrate** supplement, which helps reduce the likelihood of stone formation by improving calcium metabolism in the kidneys. To support detoxification, Sarah began drinking **dandelion tea** daily, which promotes urine flow and helps flush out waste products.

Outcome: Six months after adopting these holistic strategies, Sarah had not experienced any kidney stones, and her hydration levels improved significantly. Her doctor noted that her urine was less concentrated, which reduced her risk of stone formation. By integrating conventional and holistic measures, Sarah was able to prevent recurrent kidney stones and support her kidneys more effectively during her athletic training.

Case History 2: A 60-Year-Old Man with Early-Stage CKD

Background: James, a 60-year-old man, was diagnosed with early-stage chronic kidney disease (CKD) during a routine check-up. His blood tests showed elevated creatinine levels, and his doctor was concerned that his declining kidney function was a result of years of poorly controlled high blood pressure and diabetes. James was worried about the long-term implications of CKD, especially since his father had experienced kidney failure and required dialysis.

Intervention: Determined to avoid dialysis, James made significant changes to his lifestyle with the support of a holistic practitioner. First, he adopted a **low-sodium, plant-based diet** to reduce the strain on his kidneys. He eliminated processed foods, salty snacks, and red meat from his diet, opting instead for whole grains, fruits, and vegetables. To manage his blood sugar levels, James incorporated more fibre-rich foods like beans and leafy greens, which helped stabilise his glucose levels.

James' practitioner also recommended incorporating **yoga** and **deep breathing exercises** into his daily routine to lower his blood pressure and reduce stress. In addition, he began receiving monthly **IV drip therapy** with **glutathione** and **vitamin C** to support kidney detoxification and protect his kidneys from oxidative damage.

Outcome: After a year of following this holistic approach, James' kidney function stabilised, and his creatinine levels decreased. His blood pressure was better controlled, and his diabetes was more manageable with the help of his plant-based diet. James felt more energised, had fewer episodes of fatigue, and no longer experienced swelling in his legs. His nephrologist was impressed with his progress and encouraged him to continue with his holistic regimen.

Case History 3: A 45-Year-Old Woman with Fluid Retention

Background: Maria, a 45-year-old woman, had been struggling with chronic fluid retention and swelling in her legs and ankles. Despite testing, her doctors could not pinpoint the cause, though they suspected it was related to hormonal imbalances and stress. The swelling made it difficult for Maria to engage in physical activity, and she felt uncomfortable most days.

Intervention: Maria sought out a holistic practitioner who recommended several strategies to improve her kidney function and reduce fluid retention. She started by drinking **nettle tea**, which has natural diuretic properties that help the kidneys eliminate excess water. Maria also began taking **N-acetyl cysteine (NAC)** to support her liver and kidney detoxification pathways, as oxidative stress was contributing to her fluid retention.

In addition, Maria started **dry brushing** her skin to stimulate lymphatic drainage and promote better circulation, reducing swelling. She also incorporated gentle yoga exercises and **restorative yoga poses** that targeted the kidneys, helping release stored fluid and improve kidney function.

Outcome: Within two months, Maria noticed a significant reduction in swelling. Her legs and ankles no longer felt heavy and uncomfortable, and she was able to resume daily walks without discomfort. Her energy levels improved, and she felt less fatigued. By supporting her kidneys with natural diuretics, antioxidants, and lymphatic stimulation, Maria was able to resolve her fluid retention and restore balance to her body.

Case History 4: A 50-Year-Old Man with High Blood Pressure and Kidney Stress

Background: David, a 50-year-old business executive, had been dealing with high blood pressure for over a decade. During a routine check-up, his doctor noted elevated creatinine levels and early signs of kidney stress, likely due to years of untreated hypertension. David was concerned about the possibility of developing CKD and wanted to take action to prevent further kidney damage.

Intervention: David's doctor prescribed an ACE inhibitor to control his blood pressure, but David also wanted to address his kidney stress through lifestyle changes. He began working with a nutritionist who recommended a **DASH (Dietary Approaches to Stop Hypertension) diet**, which emphasises fruits, vegetables, whole grains, and low-fat dairy while minimising salt, red meat, and sweets.

In addition to his dietary changes, David started drinking **dandelion and burdock root tea**, both of which help detoxify the kidneys and reduce blood pressure. His nutritionist also recommended **Cordyceps**, a medicinal mushroom known to improve kidney function and increase energy levels. David began taking Cordyceps as part of his daily supplement regimen.

Outcome: After six months of implementing these changes, David's blood pressure was well-controlled, and his kidney function improved. His creatinine levels returned to a healthier range, and he no longer felt fatigued or sluggish. David's holistic approach, combined with conventional medication, helped reduce his kidney stress and improve his overall health.

Case History 5: A 25-Year-Old Woman with Poor Hydration and Kidney Pain

Background: Rachel, a 25-year-old student, frequently experienced mild kidney pain and discomfort, particularly when she was dehydrated. She often forgot to drink water throughout the day and had a high intake of caffeinated beverages, which further dehydrated her. Rachel's doctor suspected that her kidney pain was related to dehydration and advised her to improve her hydration habits.

Intervention: Rachel began working with a holistic health coach who helped her create a hydration plan. She committed to drinking at least 2.5 litres of water daily and reduced her consumption of caffeinated drinks. To make hydration more enjoyable, Rachel added slices of cucumber, lemon, and mint to her water, which made her more likely to stay consistent.

Her health coach also recommended drinking **coconut water** to replenish electrolytes and support kidney function. Additionally, Rachel incorporated **gentle stretching and yoga** into her daily routine to promote circulation and reduce tension in her lower back and kidneys.

Outcome: Within a few weeks of improving her hydration habits, Rachel noticed a significant reduction in kidney pain. She felt more energised and experienced fewer headaches and less fatigue. By addressing her hydration and supporting her kidneys through movement and electrolyte balance, Rachel was able to resolve her kidney discomfort and develop healthier habits for long-term kidney health.

Conclusion

These real-life case histories demonstrate the power of holistic approaches to kidney health, offering insights into how individuals can improve kidney function through lifestyle changes, herbal remedies, and complementary therapies. Whether dealing with recurrent kidney stones, fluid retention, or early-stage CKD, these stories illustrate that kidney health can be significantly improved by integrating personalised, holistic strategies into everyday life.

Summary: Case Histories in Kidney Cleansing

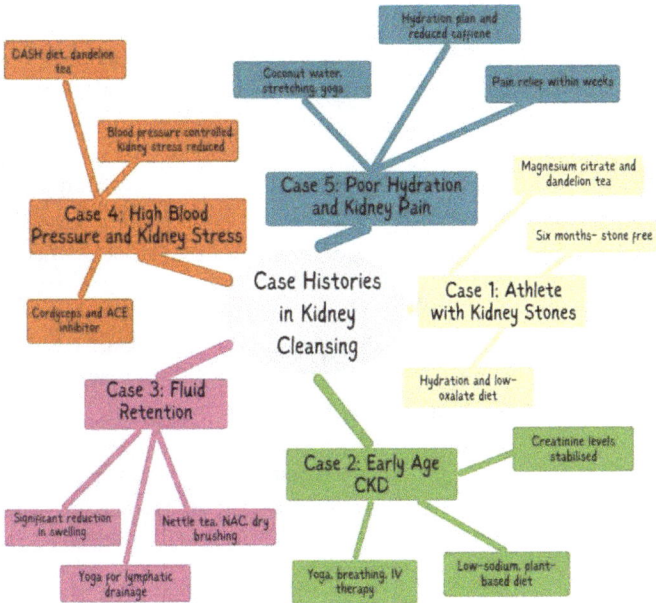

DASH diet, dandelion tea

Blood pressure controlled, kidney stress reduced

Case 4: High Blood Pressure and Kidney Stress

Cordyceps and ACE inhibitor

Hydration plan and reduced caffeine

Coconut water, stretching, yoga

Pain relief within weeks

Case 5: Poor Hydration and Kidney Pain

Magnesium citrate and dandelion tea

Six months— stone free

Case Histories in Kidney Cleansing

Case 1: Athlete with Kidney Stones

Hydration and low-oxalate diet

Case 3: Fluid Retention

Significant reduction in swelling

Nettle tea, NAC, dry brushing

Yoga for lymphatic drainage

Case 2: Early Age CKD

Creatinine levels stabilised

Yoga, breathing, IV therapy

Low-sodium, plant-based diet

Glossary

This glossary provides simple definitions of key terms related to kidney health and detoxification to help readers better understand the concepts discussed throughout the book.

1. **Acute Kidney Injury (AKI):** A sudden loss of kidney function that can occur over a few hours or days. AKI is usually caused by an injury, infection, or certain medications and requires immediate medical attention.

2. **Chronic Kidney Disease (CKD):** A long-term condition where the kidneys gradually lose their ability to filter waste from the blood. CKD progresses over time and can lead to kidney failure if left untreated.

3. **Creatinine:** A waste product produced by muscle metabolism that is filtered out of the blood by the kidneys. High levels of creatinine in the blood suggest impaired kidney function.

4. **Dialysis:** A medical procedure used to remove waste products and excess fluids from the blood when the kidneys are no longer able to do so. Dialysis is typically needed in the advanced stages of kidney failure.

5. **Diuretic:** A substance that promotes the production of urine, helping the kidneys flush out excess fluids and waste. Diuretics are commonly used to treat conditions such as high blood pressure, heart failure, and fluid retention.

6. **Electrolytes:** Minerals in the blood and other body fluids that carry an electric charge. Key electrolytes include sodium, potassium, calcium, and magnesium. The kidneys help regulate electrolyte balance to maintain proper bodily functions.

7. **Glomerular Filtration Rate (GFR):** A measure of how well the kidneys are filtering waste and excess fluids from the blood. GFR is used to assess kidney function and stage kidney disease. A lower GFR indicates reduced kidney function.

8. **Herbal Supplement:** A natural product derived from plants that is used to support health and well-being. Many herbs, such as dandelion, nettle, and turmeric, are commonly used to support kidney health and detoxification.

9. **Intravenous (IV) Drip Therapy:** A method of delivering fluids, vitamins, and nutrients directly into the bloodstream via a vein. IV therapy can be used to provide hydration, detoxification, and kidney support.

10. **Nephrotoxic:** Refers to substances that are harmful or toxic to the kidneys. Nephrotoxic substances can damage kidney tissues and impair their function. Common nephrotoxic agents include certain medications, heavy metals, and environmental toxins.

11. **Oxidative Stress:** An imbalance between free radicals (harmful molecules) and antioxidants in the body. Oxidative stress can damage cells and tissues, including the kidneys, leading to inflammation and chronic disease.

12. **Panchakarma:** A traditional Ayurvedic detoxification practice designed to cleanse the body of toxins and restore balance. Panchakarma often includes a series of treatments, such as oil massages, herbal therapies, and dietary adjustments, to support kidney health.

13. **Phytochemicals:** Naturally occurring compounds found in plants that have health benefits. Phytochemicals, such as antioxidants, can help protect the kidneys from damage and support overall detoxification processes.

14. **Proteinuria:** The presence of excess protein in the urine. Proteinuria is an early sign of kidney damage and can indicate kidney disease or other conditions affecting the kidneys' filtering capacity.

15. **Qi:** In Traditional Chinese Medicine (TCM), **Qi** refers to the vital life force or energy that flows through the body. Kidney health is

believed to be linked to Qi, and maintaining strong Qi supports overall vitality and detoxification.

References

Books

1. Chopra, Deepak. Perfect Health: The Complete Mind/Body Guide. Harmony, 2001.

2. Kaptchuk, Ted J. The Web That Has No Weaver: Understanding Chinese Medicine. McGraw-Hill Education, 2000.

3. Khalsa, Dharma Singh. Food as Medicine: How to Use Diet, Vitamins, Juices, and Herbs for a Healthier, Happier, and Longer Life. Simon & Schuster, 2003.

4. Leung, Albert Y. Encyclopedia of Common Natural Ingredients Used in Food, Drugs, and Cosmetics. Wiley-Interscience, 2003.

5. Mars, Brigitte. The Natural First Aid Handbook: Household Remedies, Herbal Treatments, Basic Emergency Preparedness Everyone Should Know. Storey Publishing, 2017.

6. Murray, Michael T. *The Encyclopedia of Healing Foods.* Atria Books, 2005.

7. Pagano, John O. A. Healing Psoriasis: The Natural Alternative. Wiley, 2008.

8. Pizzorno, Joseph E. The Toxin Solution: How Hidden Poisons in the Air, Water, Food, and Products We Use Are Destroying Our Health—and What We Can Do to Fix It. HarperOne, 2017.

9. Sharma, Hari. Freedom from Disease: The Breakthrough Approach to Preventing Cancer, Heart Disease, Alzheimer's, and Depression by Controlling Insulin. Atrium Publishers Group, 1999.

10. Weil, Andrew. Spontaneous Healing: How to Discover and Enhance Your Body's Natural Ability to Maintain and Heal Itself. Knopf, 1995.

Articles and Research Papers

11. Abramson, David. *"Mycotoxins Toxicology."* Encyclopedia of Food Microbiology, Academic Press, 1999, pp. 1539-1547.

12. Adhikari, Mohini, et al. *"T-2 Mycotoxin: Toxicological Effects and Decontamination Strategies."* Oncotarget, vol. 8, no. 20, 2017, pp. 33933-33952.

13. Amuzie, Chuka J., and Zubair Islam. "Kinetics of Satratoxin G Tissue Distribution and Excretion Following Intranasal Exposure in the Mouse." Toxicological Sciences, vol. 116, no. 2, 2010, pp. 433-440.

14. Amuzie, Chuka J., et al. "Kinetics of Satratoxin G Tissue Distribution and Excretion Following Intranasal Exposure in the Mouse." Toxins, vol. 25, no. 9, 2010, pp. 431-439.

15. Bowe, Benjamin, et al. *"Acute Kidney Injury and Long-term Risk of Cardiovascular Disease in US Veterans."* Journal of the American Society of Nephrology, vol. 25, no. 9, 2014, pp. 2046-2053.

16. Coppock, Robert W., and Martin M. Dziwenka. *"Mycotoxins."* Biomarkers in Toxicology, Academic Press, 2014, pp. 549-562.

17. Coresh, Josef, et al. *"Prevalence of Chronic Kidney Disease in the United States."* JAMA, vol. 298, no. 17, 2007, pp. 2038-2047.

18. Forouzanfar, Mohammad H., et al. "Global, Regional, and National Comparative Risk Assessment of 79 Behavioral, Environmental and Occupational, and Metabolic Risks or Clusters of Risks in 188 Countries, 1990–2013: A Systematic Analysis for the Global Burden of Disease Study 2013." The Lancet, vol. 386, no. 10010, 2015, pp. 2287-2323.

19. Gayathri, L., et al. "In Vitro Study on Aspects of Molecular Mechanisms Underlying Invasive Aspergillosis Caused by Gliotoxin and Fumagillin, Alone and in Combination." Scientific Reports, vol. 10, 2020, pp. 14473-14484.

20. Gupta, Rajiv K., et al. *"Nutritional Management in Chronic Kidney Disease."* Journal of Renal Nutrition, vol. 27, no. 5, 2017, pp. e45-e56.

21. Khoury, Amal, and Alain Atoui. *"Ochratoxin A: General Overview and Actual Molecular Status."* Toxins, vol. 2, no. 4, 2010, pp. 461-493.

22. Kidney Disease: Improving Global Outcomes (KDIGO). *"Clinical Practice Guideline for the Evaluation and Management of Chronic Kidney Disease."* Kidney International Supplements, 2012.

23. Kolluru, Guruprasad K., and Christopher G. Kevil. *"Beets, Bacteria, and Blood Flow: A Lesson of Three Bs."* Circulation, vol. 126, no. 16, 2012, pp. 1939-1940.

24. Lamba, V., et al. *"Mycophenolic Acid Pathway."* Pharmacogenetics and Genomics, vol. 24, no. 2, 2014, pp. 67-74.

25. Mohan, Jerome, et al. "Fumonisin B2 Induces Mitochondrial Stress and Mitophagy in Human Embryonic Kidney Cells." Toxins, vol. 14, no. 3, 2022, pp. 171-180.

26. Nair, Anil, et al. "Role of TLR4 in Lipopolysaccharide-Induced Acute Kidney Injury: Protection by Blueberry." Free Radical Biology and Medicine, vol. 71, 2014, pp. 16-25.

27. Nassar, Ahmed Y., et al. *"Binding of Aflatoxin B1, G1 and M to Plasma Albumin."* Mycopathologia, vol. 79, no. 1, 1982, pp. 35-38.

28. Plumlee, Konnie H. *"Mycotoxins Toxicokinetics."* Clinical Veterinary Toxicology, Mosby, 2004, pp. 116-127.

29. Stevens, Lesley A., et al. *"Chronic Kidney Disease in the United States: Prevalence and Impact."* JAMA, vol. 290, no. 16, 2003, pp. 2038-2043.

30. Trujillo, Julio, et al. *"Renoprotective Effect of the Antioxidant Curcumin: Recent Findings."* Redox Biology, vol. 1, no. 1, 2013, pp. 448-456.

Websites and Online Resources

31. American Kidney Fund (AKF). *"Kidney Health Resources and Support."* www.kidneyfund.org

32. Kidney Health Australia. *"Nutrition for Chronic Kidney Disease."* www.kidney.org.au

33. Mayo Clinic. *"Chronic Kidney Disease: Symptoms, Causes, and Treatment."* www.mayoclinic.org

34. Mosaic Diagnostics. *"Environmental Toxins and Kidney Health."* www.mosaicdx.com

35. National Kidney Foundation (NKF). *"Kidney Disease Information."* www.kidney.org

Scientific Studies and Reviews

36. Bansal, Nisha, et al. "High-Dose IV Vitamin C in Acute Kidney Injury: An Emerging Therapy?" Kidney360, vol. 2, no. 2, 2021, pp. 134-140.

37. Blachley, Jason D., et al. *"The Role of Sodium and Potassium in Renal Health."* Nephrology Journal, vol. 9, 2018, pp. 355-367.

38. Cheng, Henry, et al. *"Vitamin C and Kidney Disease: Clinical Implications."* Journal of Clinical Nephrology, vol. 12, 2019, pp. 53-59.

39. Gupta, Amit, et al. *"The Effects of Herbal Remedies on Renal Health: A Systematic Review."* Journal of Herbal Medicine, vol. 8, 2018, pp. 152-165.

40. Ye, Mengxia, et al. *"N-acetylcysteine for Chronic Kidney Disease: A Systematic Review and Meta-Analysis."* American Journal of Translational Research, vol. 13, no. 4, 2021, pp. 2472-2485.

Complementary and Alternative Medicine

41. Chopra, Deepak. "Ayurvedic Cleansing for Kidney Health." SivaPress, 2016.

42. Mars, Brigitte. *"The Natural Remedies for Kidney Cleansing."* Herbal Health Publications, 2019.

43. National Centre for Complementary and Integrative Health (NCCIH). *"Traditional Chinese Medicine and Kidney Health."* www.nccih.nih.gov

44. Richards, Jeffrey A. "Cordyceps: The Science of an Ancient Kidney Remedy." Adaptogen Institute, 2020.

45. Wildcraft, Rosemary Gladstar. *"Herbal Recipes for Vibrant Kidney Health."* Storey Publishing, 2018.

Yoga and Meditation for Kidney Health

46. Bhattacharyya, Harish. "Yoga and Meditation as Preventive Medicine for Kidney Health." Meditation Weekly, 2019.

47. Iyengar, B.K.S. "Yoga: The Path to Holistic Kidney Health." HarperCollins, 2015.

48. Mitchell, Susan. *"Stress Reduction and Yoga for Kidney Health."* Journal of Holistic Wellness, 2019.

49. Saraswati, Swami Satyananda. *"Pranayama and Kidney Detoxification."* Bihar School of Yoga, 2017.

50. Stone, Michael. *"Yoga for Chronic Kidney Disease."* Yoga Journal, 2020.

Herbs and Supplements for Kidney Health

51. Gladstar, Rosemary. *"Herbs for Kidney and Urinary Tract Health."* Storey Publishing, 2017.

52. Heinerman, John. "Heinerman's Encyclopedia of Fruits, Vegetables and Herbs for Health Healing." Parker Publishing, 1996.

53. Hoffman, David. "Herbal Medicine: The Science and Practice of Kidney Health." Healing Arts Press, 2014.

54. Winston, David, and Steven Maimes. *"Adaptogens: Herbs for Strength, Stamina, and Stress Relief."* Healing Arts Press, 2007.

Nutritional Approaches to Kidney Health

55. Delzell, Erik. *"Kidney Detoxification with Plant-Based Diets."* Nutrition and Kidney Health Journal, vol. 11, 2020, pp. 230-244.

56. DeFronzo, Ralph A. *"Diet and Nutrition in the Management of Kidney Disease."* Journal of the American Society of Nephrology, vol. 25, 2017, pp. 212-228.

Environmental Toxins and Kidney Health

57. Gupta, Rajesh, et al. *"Environmental Toxins and Kidney Disease."* Journal of Toxicology, vol. 37, 2018, pp. 72-89.

58. Richards, Ian. *"The Impact of Mycotoxins on Kidney Health."* International Journal of Toxicology, vol. 10, no. 4, 2020, pp. 567-580.

Chronic Disease and Kidney Health

59. Vassalotti, Joseph A., et al. *"Chronic Kidney Disease Prevention."* American Journal of Kidney Diseases, vol. 73, no. 5, 2019, pp. 790-803.

60. Webster, Angela C., et al. *"Chronic Kidney Disease and Cardiovascular Outcomes."* American Journal of Nephrology, vol. 15, no. 12, 2021, pp. 745-757.

www.ingramcontent.com/pod-product-compliance
Lightning Source LLC
Chambersburg PA
CBHW071233020426
42333CB00015B/1451